Scalpel, Scope, and Stain

Noah Pardell

Scalpel, Scope, and Stain

A Pathologist's Journey into Diagnostics

Springer

Noah Pardell
Department of Laboratory Medicine and Pathology
University of Alberta
Edmonton, AB, Canada

ISBN 978-3-032-25383-5 ISBN 978-3-032-25384-2 (eBook)
https://doi.org/10.1007/978-3-032-25384-2

This Springer imprint is published by the registered company Springer Nature Switzerland AG
The registered company address is: Gewerbestrasse 11, 6330 Cham, Switzerland

To my mom, who always encouraged my writing.

Competing Interests The author has no competing interests to declare that are relevant to the content of this manuscript.

Contents

About the Author

Dr. Noah Pardell is a physician, educator, and lifelong learner whose journey in medicine reflects a passion for both the sciences and the arts. He earned his BSc Honours degree in Neuroscience from the University of Alberta in 2018, followed by his Doctor of Medicine (MD) at the same institution in 2022. He is currently a PGY-5 resident in Diagnostic and Molecular Pathology (formerly Anatomical Pathology) at the University of Alberta, in Edmonton, Canada.

Noah comes from a large and diverse family, with five siblings who each have carved their own unique paths. Growing up, Noah cultivated a love for music, completing the Royal Conservatory of Music curriculum in piano, and has always enjoyed social activities and sports such as rugby and golf—especially when surrounded by friends. He is equally at home in collaborative settings and in solo pursuits, whether catching up on the latest movies or diving into a good book.

A writer at heart, Noah has consistently found joy in documenting and reflecting on his experiences, blending narrative storytelling with scientific curiosity. His interests in computer science and technology have seamlessly integrated into his medical training—culminating in projects that make complex pathology concepts more accessible through digital tools.

Noah is inspired by teamwork, intellectual challenge, and compassionate patient care. As he advances through the 5-year Diagnostic and Molecular Pathology program at the University of Alberta, he is preparing for fellowship training in Bone and Soft Tissue Pathology—a field he finds both complex and deeply rewarding. He looks forward to contributing to diagnostic medicine and pathology education, ever guided by a spirit of curiosity, empathy, and collaboration.

1 Introduction

Pathology is a hidden profession. While surgeons operate in gleaming theaters and internists make their daily rounds through bustling wards, pathologists work behind closed doors, peering into microscopes at the very building blocks of life and disease. Radiologists may see contrasting shades of grey and shadows of illness on their screens, but only the pathologist dares to pronounce definitive diagnoses based on a few cells or millimetres of tissue, often determining a patient's fate in the process. The surgeon presides over the careful dissection of a patient's anatomy, while the internist's domain encompasses medical diagnosis and treatment with pharmacologic agents. But it is the diseases themselves and their effects at the cellular and molecular level that ultimately drive the clinical symptoms these specialties encounter. The diagnosis and understanding of disease processes at all levels, both those warranting surgery and those requiring other treatments, is the purview of the pathologist.

Pathology is the study of disease. More precisely, it is the study and diagnosis of disease processes at the molecular and cellular levels. Aberrations of cellular structure or function have a bottom-up effect, culminating in altered function of the tissues the cells belong to, of the organs the tissues belong to, and ultimately the patient's overall presentation. Conversely, the signs and symptoms a patient presents with are reflections of diseases and their mechanisms at these lower levels. The interesting thing is that many diseases

N. Pardell, *Scalpel, Scope, and Stain*,
https://doi.org/10.1007/978-3-032-25384-2_1

produce visible changes in the cells and tissues that can be seen through a microscope. The pathologist has the opportunity to voyage beyond what is seen with the naked eye into a realm most people and even other physicians have not been to, nor understand the soil it is made up of.

The daily practice of a pathologist is varied, from examining biopsy material or surgically resected organ tissues, performing autopsies to elucidate causes of death, teaching other medical professionals, collaborating on challenging cases, and sometimes engaging in research activities. It is a medical specialty that is rewarding, challenging, and that affords a work-life balance few others can rival.

There is a misconception about pathology being a profession disconnected from patients. Although the pathologist usually (but not always) operates within the confines of their office, does not routinely run a clinic, and does not wake up at five in the morning to review patient charts on the ward, they play an integral but overlooked role in patient care.

The process of working through a patient case involves an amalgamation of a patient's history, their blood test results, progress notes from other physicians, nurses, and other medical professionals, as well as radiologic reports and prior pathology reports. It is then that, in the context of the individual patient, an accurate diagnosis can be made. In fact, the pathology report is the primary driver for what happens next in a patient's course through the medical system. Calling something cancerous or *malignant* when in fact it is relatively innocuous or *benign*, can mean the difference between giving the patient a couple of doses of a drug versus a risky operation, potentially with chemotherapy and radiation, all with a plethora of side effects. This demonstrates the double-edged sword of pathology—due to the critical nature of having to be as certain as possible with your diagnoses, the price the patient could pay for an error is profound. It is thus a very common practice among pathologists to collaborate and ask for opinions on particularly challenging cases, which helps illustrate the interpersonal skills that pathologists exercise.

Pathologists do not work in isolation. I believe one of the deterring factors for medical students not choosing pathology other than a lack of knowledge about the specialty (which this book aims to address), is the assumption that pathologists do not like people, work in a basement and prefer the dead to the living. Speaking for myself, this is not true. Pathologists may not directly interact with patients very much, but they are constantly interacting with colleagues, other physicians, and laboratory staff to render correct diagnoses and direct a patient's treatment course. It is not uncommon for a pathologist to directly call other clinicians or securely chat with them to tell them about an unexpected finding in their patient's biopsy or surgical resection specimen, especially if it is time sensitive. As for the work environment, the pathologist is not on the ward looking at vital signs and scribbling progress notes on the patient's chart only for their pager to beep and interrupt their workflow because they have to manage an incoming trauma in the emergency department, all within 30 min of their 26-h *consecutive* in-house call shift. Those experiences were exciting in medical school and the first year of residency, but I can proudly say that I would much prefer to sit in my well-lit room playing house music and taking a sip out of my third coffee for the day while analyzing glass slides of a patient's esophagus for any spurious cancer cells still alive after being bombarded with radiation and chemotherapy.

The goal of this book is to shine a light on a medical specialty that is often overlooked and to illustrate the important place that Anatomical Pathology has within the medical specialty milieu. This book is intended to cater to medical students but should be readily accessible to anyone interested in the inner workings of medicine and pathology. I will illustrate my own journey into pathology and my understanding of this fascinating specialty as it stands at the present day. In doing so, I hope to convey the essential nature of pathology and laboratory medicine as well as diagnostic medicine at large. I hope to inform the next generation of medical students looking towards the future, and to demystify the workings, challenges, and triumphs of a pathologist's day-to-day work, as I believe the allure of the specialty requires a vicarious retelling of real cases, diagnostic dilemmas, problem-solving, and their solutions. How else can you truly appreciate something without feeling as though you are looking through the eyes of those in the shoes you might hope to fill?

The details regarding patient cases, particularly their clinical histories, have been altered and elements selectively fictionalized to maintain patient confidentiality and maintain ethical integrity. However, being based on the real cases, such changes do not alter the plausibility of the presentations nor detract from the insights and experiences regarding them.

Suggested Readings

1. College of American Pathologists [Internet]. [cited 2026 Feb 9]. What is pathology? https://www.cap.org/member-resources/articles/what-is-pathology
2. Funkhouser WK. Pathology: the clinical description of human disease. In: Essential concepts in molecular pathology. Amsterdam, The Netherlands: Academic Press; 2020. p. 177–90.
3. Mayer C. Understanding stigma and public perception of pathology: a public relations perspective. Acad Pathol. 2025;12(4):100226.

2 A Microscopic Trap

I did not plan on entering Anatomical Pathology when I started medical school. With my undergraduate degree in Neuroscience and my enjoyment of learning human anatomy, 22-year-old me thought that I had to be a surgeon; originally, a neurosurgeon to be specific. The tunnel vision was far-reaching, precluding me from truly investigating other specialties with an open mind. Throughout medical school, I would take some time when I was not studying to observe the surgeons in their natural habitat, the operating room, known as *shadowing*. The allure built upon itself whenever I saw the scalpel transgress the skin's barrier at the start of every case. Later on, I had some elective time I used to explore the specialty at home and at other institutions, where I did more than just shadow; I assisted staff neurosurgeons during brain tumour operations, got to drill burr-holes in patient's skulls to access the brain, and hurriedly sutured a man's scalp back together after a major trauma incident. It wasn't until the end of my third year of medical school (which is a 4-year program in North America) that my vision of my career path started to change.

I was on an away rotation at a community hospital for obstetrics and gynecology, the specialty dealing with all things related to women, the reproductive process, birth, and labour. On a peculiarly slow shift, the junior resident and I started to chat about my future. I told him my aim was to become a surgeon. He told me he used to be

N. Pardell, *Scalpel, Scope, and Stain*,
https://doi.org/10.1007/978-3-032-25384-2_2

in surgery but opted to switch residency programs after he and his siblings saw the effect it was having on him mentally and physically. An internal struggle ensued; continue this career without regard to personal satisfaction and wellness, or switch specialties, change future plans, and potentially find a better fit for his personality. He chose the latter.

The stories he told me chipped away at the notions and stereotypes I held too much on a pedestal about the day-to-day life of some specialties. He told me stories during his first year practicing in a particular specialty of surgery of sleepless nights, extreme anxiety, and sometimes seemingly little support from superiors. He described frequent harrowing incidents and illustrated the reality of spending days *in* the hospital without seeing his significant other. He described the hidden curriculum of medicine, where resident wellness protocols that are put in place by the health organization are frowned upon in an unspoken manner. For example, after a standard 26 h shift in some clinical specialties on in-house call (where you live in the hospital managing patients as well as operate through the night if rotating on surgery), you are entitled for a 'post-call' day, where the idea is that you get to go home after reviewing what events and situations happened that night with the daytime team and recuperate until you get back to work the following morning. As well, there are limits on how many call shifts you can do in a month. These were usually only treated as guidelines in some surgical and non-surgical specialties with high volumes. And it was a similar story I heard from other residents in other programs at various locations.

Leaving after 26 h was seen as a weakness, or even selfishness, due to removing yourself from the pool of doctors to help manage the ever-busy wards. People will frequently stay long past 26 h (sometimes working the full post-call day) to clock around 36 h in 2 days. This is the unfortunate reality of many medical specialties to this day, although seemingly more prominent in surgical specialties, despite major improvements having been made. It is interesting that for many, to become a doctor and steward of health, you must become very unhealthy yourself. This culture is slowly improving (as any systemic change does), with many stewards of change hailing from the surgical ranks themselves.

I can recount another conversation with a staff pediatric surgeon during a meet-and-greet event at an international conference, whereby I inquired as to the day-to-day life taking care of children and adolescents in a specialty fraught with danger. Staring at the ground, with weariness and despondence, she proclaimed four words that should have been my cue to scrupulously evaluate my aspirations: 'It takes your life.'

I have heard stories of doctors hallucinating in operating rooms due to sleep deprivation. I have had other resident physicians boast about how many renal lithotripsy procedures they have undergone (a non-surgical treatment for kidney and ureter stones whereby high-energy shock waves are transmitted through the body to break down and reduce the stones into smaller pieces, allowing passage through the urine), due to never having time to drink water—a major risk factor for forming such stones being dehydration. They wore these adverse health outcomes as badges of honour rather than seeing them as ill omens of a career that tends to take rather than give, especially if you are not adamant on prioritizing yourself.

It is important to recognize, however, that many people thrive in these environments. The high-intensity pacing and the never-ending demand to improve one's surgical skill and aptitude are exactly what future surgeons use to fuel their tenacious drive and reach their full potential. The camaraderie and the immediate impact the profession has on patients are unparalleled. In fact, many of my close friends are in surgical specialties, and I admire them and what they practice, deeply valuing their contributions to improving patients' lives and always acting in their patients' best interests. Many of the people I know would choose the specialty all over again, highlighting that my experiences and perspectives are not universal, but simply a personal account. Nobody knows yourself better than you, so it is incumbent upon you to assess your future aspirations on your terms alone. By shadowing, doing electives, asking to see the variety of roles a resident and staff do behind the scenes, and reading others' medical narratives (such as this one), you will find the right fit for your personality and circumstances.

These descriptions and experiences are extolled for the main purpose of encouraging future physicians to avoid the mistake that I made; namely, to keep an open mind about possible personality fit with the realities of the job, regardless of the specialty they have in their sights. I also convey these experiences not to discourage future surgeons from the vocation they may feel compelled to explore, but to inform those whose surgical experiences do not reach past the operating room into the practical, the bread-and-butter, and the emotional encumbrance that is inexplicably inherent to such specialties. I impart these experiences not as a warning against applying to these specialties—they are, in fact, pathology's main customers and whose patients require our servitude and expertise—but as a juxtaposition to the culture of pathology. All medical training requires sacrifices of time, energy, and money. They also challenge the emotional resilience of those who undergo such training, albeit in different forms. I now believe it is imperative to fully examine all specialties rather than letting tunnel vision dictate your future. Only with open eyes can you commit to a specialty and not resent it in the future due to the challenges it imparts upon you.

After harbouring some doubt as to if surgery was for me, I switched my gaze to plastic surgery, as I did not want to give up operative experience, and this was a specialty that allowed me to specialize, in the future, in peripheral nerve surgery. This topic was very intriguing to me, motivating me to do electives in anatomy, dissecting cadavers to follow the median, ulnar, and radial nerves as they course down the upper extremity and innervate a complex of muscles. I wrote an article that was published in *PRS Global Open* and opted to be on call almost daily throughout my plastic surgery electives across Canada to gain exposure to the specialty, but also to market myself as a passionate and serious candidate for the position. At one point, my residence was located over 30 min from the hospital I was working at, and despite not having any accommodations for medical students on-call, I heard rumours that it was an unspoken expectation that you were always available to help and show your zeal for the specialty should they need assistance overnight. Whether this was true or not, I hedged my bets and figured that, should I be called for an emergent case, it would not look favourable to say 'I'll be right there, just give me *forty* minutes to get there.' I thus converted my SUV in the parking lot into a queen bed, sleeping just outside the hospital in case I got called or *paged*. I booked hotel rooms near the hospital for the same reason.

Eventually, it was time for the CaRMS match (Canadian Residency Matching Service), a system set up to allow programs at different universities across Canada to rank applicants as well as each fourth-year medical student to rank their preferred specialty and location for residency. If this process was a poker game, I went all-in. I applied widely across Canada to only plastic surgery, believing that this was the only thing I wanted to do that would give me a feeling of fulfilment, despite the stories and wisdom gleaned from my foray into neurosurgery the first 3 years of medical school. At the time, the COVID-19 pandemic was in full swing, and it was expected that most students would only match at their home program due to not being allowed to rotate or do electives at outside institutions (to minimize travel and thus prevent the spread of the virus). The true machinations of the CaRMS algorithm remain a mystery, but just as suspected, I got one interview at my home program.

When the time for 'the match' was upon my medical school cohort, I was anxious yet hopeful. I would be a plastic surgeon, I said to myself, and nothing would sway my confidence in that. However, it was not to be; I did not match in the first round. My future aspirations were shattered. However, before I could fully grieve my reality, the list of all specialties that still had openings was released for the second (and last) round of CaRMS that year. Most of the specialties listed were non-surgical specialties, a group of specialties I never once gave an honest assessment of, nor allowed myself to percolate their potential for fulfilment and purpose in my life. Among these specialties was Anatomical Pathology. Given the short time to explore these specialties as well as get three new letters of reference (for a discipline I did not have the foggiest notion as to its role in medicine), I hurriedly devoured any information I could on this specialty that had the root word 'anatomy,' as the anatomical dissections in medical school intrigued me and I thoroughly enjoyed knowing the intimate relationships of structures coursing through the body. I quickly researched, miraculously got letters of reference, and applied. I got an interview. Some time later, I received the email: I had matched to Anatomical Pathology.

What followed was a blur, a bittersweet experience that had my emotions crawling over one another. The feeling of relief from matching in general gave way to disappointment for not matching my original choice of surgery, which morphed into confusion as to what I had matched into. I did not do any electives in pathology, nor did I truly know the reality of what I was now on track to practice.

It was a period of happiness, sorrow, confusion, and perplexity. It was the greatest thing to ever happen to my career.

The only notion I had of pathology was on my medical school clerkship where I would look up what diagnosis the patient had from their prior surgery, erroneously concluding that pathology just "gives the answer." Pathology was this omnipotent entity that received samples and provided the truth. The only thing I knew about pathology was that they looked at pink and purple slides under a microscope and somehow interpreted meaning from the various geometric shapes. I could count on two hands how many histology slides I was exposed to, usually briefly on 1 slide during 80-slide PowerPoint lectures. Now I was venturing into the unknown, the unfamiliar, and the misunderstood. However, I was unknowingly venturing into an oasis of knowledge, of patient impact, and of intellectual satisfaction. I finally arrived at home.

Suggested Readings

1. Freeman B. The ultimate guide to choosing a medical specialty. 4th ed. New York: McGraw-Hill Education; 2019.
2. Lempp H, Seale C. The hidden curriculum in undergraduate medical education: qualitative study of medical students' perceptions of teaching. BMJ. 2004;329(7469):770–3.

3 Behind the Looking Glass

The first few months of my residency were spent at the university site, being introduced to the laboratory and the rooms in which I would be situated throughout the various rotations, or *blocks*. Walking around this environment was completely foreign to me and distinctly opposed to the chaos and clamour of the clinical wards. There were no cardiac monitors with (hopefully) normal and rhythmic beeping, no phones ringing incessantly, no hum of mechanical ventilators nor the commotion of patients leaving 'against medical advice' being fervently persuaded to stay in the hospital for their own benefit and health. There was a calmness and solitude that resounded loudly in my ears. Such a juxtaposition from the environments I was familiar with further led me into doubts as to if pathology was for me.

The resident rooms had multiple desks, each with its own *Nikon* or *Leica* microscopes as well as a computer. There were stacks of slides throughout the room, piled upon each other. The resident library consisted of longitudinally mounted shelves replete with a plethora of textbooks on every subspecialty within pathology. And best of all, there were windows, a feature that directly confronted my preconceived notions of pathology being a specialty relegated to darkness and basements.

The other residents were, and continue to be, excellent people, each with their own personality but all with a common passion and interest in the subject, which they happily, eagerly, and unabashedly

N. Pardell, *Scalpel, Scope, and Stain*,
https://doi.org/10.1007/978-3-032-25384-2_3

made crystal clear. Between impromptu informal teaching sessions and the provision of advice for the future, these were the people who helped me realize that pathology might just be where I needed to be.

I began to learn the scope of pathology after my 'off-service' years, where I rotated in other disciplines like General Surgery, Dermatology, Medical Oncology, Emergency Medicine, Radiology, Pediatrics, Internal Medicine, and Gynecology. After returning from my off-service obligations, I had a newfound understanding of work-life balance, but most importantly, that my original aspirations of clinical medicine may not have been an accurate reflection of what I truly would be happy with. I was now on pathology rotations, eager to learn its intricacies, but nervous at the possibility that it, too, would leave me dismayed. I quickly realized through 'sign out' with staff (where you review the cases assigned to you and learn from your inevitable mistakes), teaching sessions with other residents and Academic Half-Day (where half the day is spent learning through didactic or sometimes in-person sessions), that pathology had something I unknowingly craved.

I used to be called 'Mr. Q' during my undergraduate degree, infamous for asking questions and liaising with the professors after class to iron out any misunderstandings on whatever subject we were being taught. I like to know 'why' things happen and am not content with the answer that they 'just do.' I tend to operate in a reductionist fashion to my understandings of things, beginning at basic principles and, building upon this foundation, traversing upwards through higher levels of complexity until arriving at the level of understanding that is satisfactory for the question asked. Many disciplines are readily understandable this way, operating according to hierarchical organization, much like a computer. There is a similar paradigm in medicine, biology, and the study of disease states, except instead of circuit boards and transistors, there are symptoms, cells, molecular genetics, and biochemistry. Understanding diseases such as systemic lupus erythematosus or thyroid cancer is accessible to all physicians, but it is the pathologist who gets to play the part of an electrical and computer engineer, examining the lower layers and constituents from which the symptomatology the patient presents with arises from.

It was this aspect of pathology—the ability to look 'under-the-hood' at the multitude of diseases learned about in medical school—that finally enlightened me as to my true place in medicine. To function as a pathologist, you must learn things never taught to you in medical school. You must recognize *histology*, the microscopic appearance of the various cells and tissues of the body in various states of normalcy. You then gradually build up knowledge of *histopathology*, the appearance of the same tissues and cells in diseased states. This is much of the focus of pathology, the recognition of a wide variety of diseases based on patterns, cell types, interactions and interplays between and within the various tissue structures. It is this complex microenvironment that the pathologist learns to master, piecing together the tale told by the minuscule inhabitants of this foreign land in the context of the individual patient's health. The pathologist incorporates knowledge of the patient's history, radiology, and blood test results. These, combined with the epidemiology and location of lesions (how prevalent and likely a particular condition or tumour is to present in this particular age group in this particular location of the body), combined with the histologic picture under the microscope to render a *differential diagnosis*.

The differential diagnosis is the cornerstone of clinical medicine, and it is ubiquitous within pathology as well. Given the entire context of the patient's history and presentation, and what is seen under the microscope, a list of potential and likely entities and diseases is created in one's mind to guide further work-up of a case. Diseases at the top of the list are most likely, whereas those at the bottom are less likely. Such a differential list guides appropriate next steps, whether it be ordering further immunohistochemical studies on the tissue (specialized stains utilizing antibodies that attach to specific markers of interest in the tissue), molecular testing such as polymerase chain reaction (PCR) or next-generation sequencing (NGS), or other special stains. These 'ancillary studies' further narrow the list of potential suspects, and the pathologist amalgamates this information to arrive at a final diagnosis.

This sleuthing is at the core of pathology, but other essential skills are taught and built upon throughout residency training. When a surgeon takes out an organ, or *resects* it, said tissue is shuttled to the laboratory. Here, the specimen is prepared for the *gross examination*, where a Pathologists' Assistant (PA) or resident will examine it, orient it, describe it, and take pieces from it to create the slides seen under the microscope. The pertinent relationships and features of the tissue or organ being 'grossed' are dependent on the specific question and what was received.

For example, a mass residing in the kidney may have had a prior biopsy demonstrating cancer, in this example, let's say a *clear cell renal cell carcinoma*. This is a common primary malignancy of the kidney, and a usual specimen the lab might receive is from a urologic surgeon who resects the kidney in a *radical nephrectomy* operation. What is received will be the kidney with the mass, the attached ureter (the thick tube that acts as a conduit for urine made from the kidney to travel into the bladder below), and the artery and vein supplying the kidney tissue. There will also be fatty tissue surrounding the kidney (*perirenal fat*), which may or may not also contain the adrenal gland on that side (the adrenal glands sit above the kidneys within the fatty tissue). During the gross examination, the grosser will examine the specimen, take measurements and weights of the structures, and begin by taking the *margins*. A surgical margin is anywhere the surgeon had to use a scalpel or blunt dissection techniques to extract the tissues. As such, it is important to document if the margins have any evidence of cancer, as this means that there is likely residual cancer still left in the patient (the tricky thing with cancer is that sometimes there is microscopic extension of malignant cells beyond the resolution of the naked eye, and so the surgeon may seem sure they got all of the tumour, but under the microscope it extends to and presumably past the margin). Thus is the rationale for the grosser to slice the margins off the specimen to process them for microscopic examination.

Next, the grosser will measure the mass, take sections of it (including any areas that look 'different' than the surroundings) to document the type of cancer and any elements that would make the tumour higher risk for the patient. Next, sections are taken at the interface of the mass and the surrounding important structures to document any extension or *invasion* of these structures, which might change the *stage* of the tumour for the patient, affecting prognostication (likelihood of a good outcome for the patient) and even treatment options (chemotherapy etc.). In this example of a *clear cell renal cell carcinoma*, it is important to document invasion of the fatty tissue of the renal sinus, as well as extension into the renal vein (sometimes kidney cancers like to crawl up the renal vein like a snake, occasionally extending all the way into the right atrium of the heart), and the kidney capsule/perirenal fat. If there is an adrenal gland, it is important to document if the tumour directly invades the gland, or if there is a deposit of tumour that is distinct and separate from the main mass, as the latter would indicate a *metastasis*, greatly affecting the *stage* of the patient.

But sometimes there is no cancer, even when suspected. I had a case where a patient was suspected of having a mass in their cecum (the beginning of the large intestine) due to their clinical symptoms. Radiology gave a differential diagnosis of the 'mass' based on the CT scan, which included the potential that this was not a mass at all but rather just a redundant or prominent mucosal fold (normal tissue projecting into the bowel). For reasons I am not privy to, the surgeon performed a right hemicolectomy, resecting a large component of the large intestine due to their high clinical suspicion of cancer. When grossing the specimen, my attending physician and I could not find any mass or projection that could explain the clinical and radiologic findings. As such, in addition to the standard sections of margins and bowel itself, we elected to submit the cecum in its entirety, in case there was some lesion we could see microscopically. At the time of microscopic examination, all I could see was normal large bowel tissue. Thus, this patient had an erroneous right hemicolectomy to treat a cancer that did not exist. This case highlights the essential role of pathology not only in diagnosis but also in quality assurance, feeding back to other practitioners the results of their interventions. Without pathology, the patient theoretically could have gone on to undergo chemotherapy for a cancer they never had, which, as you might surmise, is unacceptable and introduces a host of side effects, notwithstanding the psychological and social implications of thinking you have cancer.

Every rotation built upon the last, developing the skills and diagnostic acumen to not only understand what it is you are looking at under the microscope, but to interpret and assess the tissues in such a manner as to yield the salient features that will determine the patient's diagnosis, treatment, and prognosis at times. The following chapter will highlight some of those diagnoses that are nefarious and crucial not to miss, but that oftentimes masquerade as seemingly innocuous and innocent. It is these examples that might keep a pathologist up at night, and those which necessitate constant vigilance by the practitioner behind the microscope.

Suggested Readings

1. Kumar V, Abbas AK, Aster JC, Debnath J, Das A. Robbins, Cotran & Kumar pathologic basis of disease. 11th ed. Philadelphia: Elsevier; 2025.
2. Pawlina, W. Histology: a text and atlas. 9th ed. Wolters Kluwer Health; 2023.
3. Tan J, Xiao X. Harness first-principles thinking in problem-based learning for chemical education. J Chem Educ. 2025;102(2):943–7. https://doi.org/10.1021/acs.jchemed.4c01178.

Wolves in Sheep's Clothing

4

In clinical medicine, there are diseases that are known as 'The Great Imitators,' insofar as their myriad symptoms and variable presentations often mimic other, usually more common, diseases. They can present with multisystem involvement and present in a large range of ways in different patients. Such notorious disease entities include syphilis, systemic lupus erythematosus, and even tuberculosis. These disease entities reside almost permanently on any differential diagnosis an internal medicine physician might construct when faced with an undifferentiated patient (a patient who needs a diagnosis to explain their symptoms and therefore guide treatment).

Similarly, in pathology, these entities are also always at the back of a pathologist's mind when seeing specific patterns of injury under the microscope. However, there are even more mimics in pathology by virtue of the pathologist being able to bear witness to the *morphology* of diseased tissues under the microscope, or how the cells look and organize themselves. Pathologist's must be ever-vigilant, especially when encountering a case with a wide differential diagnosis. This ensures patient safety and affords the patient with a correct diagnosis so that further management (and the side effects thereof) are appropriate and harm is mitigated. In being discerning, pathologist's can reduce their chances of missing a malignancy or diagnosing the wrong disease, which could result in inappropriate management of the patient. The importance of good morphologic

N. Pardell, *Scalpel, Scope, and Stain*,
https://doi.org/10.1007/978-3-032-25384-2_4

characterization, ancillary testing, and clinical and radiologic correlation in pathology cannot be overstated.

For example, I did a dermatopathology elective, the area of pathology dealing with all diseases that are inherent to the skin and its layers or involve the skin in a systemic fashion. Here I gained experience in diagnosing common skin cancers such as squamous cell carcinoma, basal cell carcinoma, as well as benign nevi ('moles') and adnexal tumours (tumours of hair follicles, sebaceous glands, etc.). In addition, there were lots of inflammatory conditions that necessitated recognition of different patterns of injury. Sometimes lymphocytes (a white blood cell that forms a major component of the immune system) react in certain ways to different disease entities. Sometimes they are surrounding the blood vessels close to the epidermis, or deeper in the dermis. Sometimes they form a confluent 'band' right beneath the epidermis without anything deeper. Sometimes the inflammatory cells aren't lymphocytes but rather neutrophils, another white blood cell that often participates in acute inflammatory reactions. Depending on the pattern of injury and cell types involved, a differential is yielded.

One day I received a skin biopsy from a patient who had a firm non-pigmented mass on their arm, with their dermatologist being concerned for a cancer. Their clinical suspicions included everything from non-melanoma skin cancer to a benign scar-like lesion known as a dermatofibroma to melanoma. Under the microscope, there was disorganized scar-like tissue in the middle of the biopsy with the surrounding epidermis (top layer of skin) looking fairly normal. There were numerous lymphoid aggregates in the dermis (a collection of lymphocytes). My first thought was that this was a dermatofibroma, possibly irritated by the patient picking at it, or just an old scar as the clinician postulated. I was ready to review with my staff this seemingly easy case. Upon review, however, they pointed out something I missed; this patient was a gravel truck driver and this lesion was on the left arm. Often, when driving long hours, professional drivers will hang their left arm out the window exposing it to sunlight, resulting in the aptly named 'trucker tan.' This means there is more ultraviolet light exposure in this area of skin, a type of radiation that is a strong driver for skin cancers due to its damaging effects on the DNA of skin cells. This was one of the features that prompted us to look closer. Upon closer inspection, the seemingly bland-looking cells forming haphazard arrangements with surrounding fibrous tissue were much darker and slightly atypical in shape than is typical of a scar or dermatofibroma. They were spindled, a term denoting that the cell shape is oblong and tapered, longer than they are wide. Still, I thought, there was no melanin pigment to suggest a melanoma, and this did not look like any melanoma I had seen to that day.

I soon learned that the morphologic differential included dermatofibroma, atypical dermatofibroma, scar tissue, neurofibroma, and *desmoplastic melanoma*. Based on the morphology, basal cell carcinoma and squamous cell carcinoma were ruled out. They just didn't look like these types of cancers. Despite this, we opted to order additional immunohistochemical stains to confirm what cells these were (squamous cells versus melanocytes versus Schwann cells in neurofibroma). CD34, a marker for vascular endothelial cells but which is helpful to interrogate tissue for other entities, was completely negative. This means the atypical cells we observed on the original section did not react to the antibody against CD34, which means that under the microscope, the cells did not stain with a brown colour. S100, a marker that stains neurofibromas and melanomas, was diffusely positive (and therefore brown). SOX10, a marker of melanocytes, was positive in all of the spindled cell nuclei. HMB-45, another marker for melanoma, however, was negative.

What we were looking at was a *desmoplastic melanoma (DM)*, a variant of melanoma that has a different clinical and microscopic appearance from conventional melanomas but also has differences in immunohistochemical and gene expression profiles, as well as biologic behaviour. It is usually *amelanotic*, or non-pigmented, a stark difference to the classic melanoma with black pigment (melanin) we commonly think about. It also often does not express all of the melanoma markers, such as this case with a negative HMB-45 stain. It mimics scars, neurofibromas, dermatofibromas, and other skin cancers. Recognition of this entity is easy to miss, but crucial for proper assessment and treatment of the patient, including their need for close follow-up to monitor recurrence of the cancer or for signs of *metastasis*—spread of the cancer to distant sites in the body. Had I been on my own (I am a resident after all), this patient may have theoretically been diagnosed with a dermatofibroma, left as is, and later presented with widespread metastases to various organs resulting in palliation and/or death.

Melanoma is not only on the differential for primary skin pathologies, but also cancers that present in organs and lymph nodes as a metastasis. We call this a 'cancer of unknown primary,' a metastatic cancer with an unknown origin site. Due to the heterogeneous nature of how melanoma can look like under the microscope, it is never a bad idea to rule it out by ordering appropriate ancillary tests like SOX10, S100, MART-1, or HMB-45. Every pathologist will have a story of a melanoma showing up in a site far removed from the skin, sometimes with a patient with no known history of melanoma, that led them on a wild goose chase to determine its identity and origin. When it is confirmed, it is usually presented to other pathologists as a warning to always keep a low threshold of suspicion for this entity.

This highlights another challenge with pathology—among the diapason of diseases and cancer types specifically, there are usually numerous *subtypes* that one must be aware of, often diverging in some way from the conventional morphologic and immunohistochemical profiles of that type. For example, among the blanket term 'colorectal adenocarcinoma,' or colon cancer, there are various subtypes, including adenoma-like, adenosquamous, carcinoma with sarcomatoid components, medullary, micropapillary, mucinous, serrated, signet ring cell, and undifferentiated subtypes. A signet ring cell adenocarcinoma of the colon can look so far removed from the adenosquamous subtype that it is hard to see that they are derived from the same epithelial cell of the intestines.

Another example of morphologic imitation can be seen with prostate biopsies. When a clinician suspects prostate cancer due to a patient's age, urinary symptoms, digital rectal examination, laboratory studies such as PSA levels, or a combination of these, they can refer to a radiologist who conducts a biopsy of the prostate gland. Under the microscope, many physiologic changes, especially with age, can be seen that can lead a pathologist to erroneously diagnosis prostatic adenocarcinoma (cancer of the prostate gland). The converse holds true too, as prostate cancer itself can sometimes look like some of these preneoplastic (not quite cancer but on its way) or benign conditions. On a particular rotation in surgical pathology in my third year of residency, I was in charge of a few prostate biopsies each week. It was not uncommon for me to mistake benign entities such as prostatic gland atrophy or basal cell hyperplasia for prostatic adenocarcinoma or high-grade prostatic intraepithelial neoplasia, respectively. I gradually learned the key features of prostate cancer that signalled its presence in the tissue over my rotation, including prominent nucleoli, rigid luminal borders, eosinophilic secretions, perineural invasion, among others. With practice, my 'hit rate' greatly improved, but one must always keep in mind the mimics. If you don't think about it, you won't see it.

Although much of pathology rests on differentiating one tumour from another (especially because many can show similar morphology), entities on a differential diagnosis for a given case are often not limited to tumours or *neoplastic* entities. Many inflammatory, autoimmune, and infectious conditions can cause diagnostic dilemmas in both radiology and pathology. Infectious diseases such as syphilis can cause syphilitic hepatitis, mimicking autoimmune hepatitis, or syphilitic proctitis causing a rectal mass that might be confused with a carcinoma or lymphoma. Tuberculosis can result in mass-like lesions of the lung known as *granulomas*, which in and of themselves have a differential diagnosis including sarcoidosis, vasculitis, rheumatoid nodules, fungal infections, etc. IgG4-related disease is a chronic, immune-mediated fibroinflammatory disorder that can mimic malignancies and infections. For example, it can imitate pancreatic cancer by forming a mass in the pancreas seen on a CT scan. The pathologist would see dense groups of IgG4-positive *plasma cells* (a type of white blood cell) with a storiform pattern of fibrosis, but no malignant/cancerous cells.

The vigilance needed to not miss important calls in pathology is the reason many pathologists triage their work so that they deal with the more complicated and uncertain cases earlier in the day when they are still 'fresh,' and leave the less critical cases and those cases which have a very limited differential to the end of the day, so as to maximize their diagnostic yield resulting in the safest practice for patients.

Throughout pathology training, you run into a plethora of tables and charts in textbooks and via online learning resources that help you differentiate diseases that all mimic each other, usually as a result of their morphology. You can find lists and tables of all cancers that exhibit a *clear cell* appearance, or those that are composed of all *small round blue cells*. Others include *spindle cell* tumours and *oncocytic* neoplasms, among many others. In addition to morphology, you can also find differential tables depicting tumours stratified based on their expression of immunohistochemical stains. As you might surmise, the list of entity types (and their subtypes) is immense, commonly overlaps, and makes for a difficult diagnostic process, especially at the beginning. However, through experience and provision of patient context, the brain begins to sift and sort these diagnoses almost unconsciously—the brain is, after all, a pattern-recognition machine—and depending on what you see under the microscope, connects the dots. The difficult part at the beginning of residency is that you must build up a foundation of knowledge for these unconscious autonomous systems to parse. This requires conscious thought, study, and feedback.

In fact, learning pathology is much like learning a new motor skill. Take playing piano, for instance, a pastime that I was fortunate enough to stick with beginning at 5 years of age. In the beginning, every movement of the fingers, the force applied to the keys to achieve a specific volume, and the coordination between the fingers on one hand as well as with those, often asynchronous, with the other hand, requires effort and conscious thought. Over time, however, these processes are shunted away from conscious awareness, freeing up space for other higher-order functions, such as foreshadowing the upcoming key change with a change in dynamics or just trying to stay at the correct tempo.

Trusting the learning process is difficult, but as with any skill, when the base building blocks are actively put into place, the rest is built upon it with a domino effect.

Every patient case requires the pathologist to construct a differential diagnosis for what they are seeing under the microscope. In fact, constructing a differential diagnosis is a vital skill for any physician regardless of specialty. The following brief discussion will illustrate two of my preferred approaches to constructing a differential I utilized during medical school clerkship and in my off-service rotations in first year residency. As noted above, pathologists take this constructed differential and carry it forward with the added information related to the morphology of the tissue under the microscope, their staining patterns, and molecular diagnostic information.

The **VITAMIN CDE mnemonic** and the **Anatomical approach** are two frameworks I have used when constructing a differential diagnosis. Each approach affords unique insights to aid a learner in systematically assessing possible causes of a condition or pathology. The VITAMIN CDE mnemonic categorizes potential diagnoses by cause (known as etiology), systematically exploring possibilities according to well-established broad categories a disease might fit into, with the understanding that some diseases span multiple categories. Each letter stands for a category: **Vascular, Infectious/Inflammatory, Traumatic/Toxic, Autoimmune/Allergic, Metabolic, Iatrogenic/Idiopathic, Neoplastic, Congenital, Degenerative, and Endocrine**. For example, in a patient presenting with jaundice, this mnemonic prompts consideration of vascular causes like ischemic hepatitis, infectious causes such as viral hepatitis, or metabolic conditions such as Gilbert's syndrome. This method ensures no major category is overlooked—which is critical when assessing patients with a complex or undifferentiated presentation.

The **Anatomical approach** organizes the differential diagnosis systematically as well, although in a different way. Following this approach, a clinician can work through possible causes by analyzing the structures that could be affected within the region of the body where the pathological process is located. As such, this spatial thinking is particularly valuable for localized symptoms, such as abdominal or chest pain. For example, in abdominal pain, one might start with the skin (e.g., herpes zoster, cellulitis, panniculitis), then proceed to deeper structures like the organs of the gastrointestinal tract (e.g., appendicitis, diverticulitis in the colon), vascular elements (e.g., mesenteric ischemia), and so forth. Similarly, for chest pain, an Emergency Medicine physician once taught me to imagine an arrow piercing through the chest to sequentially evaluate each structure it encounters—from the skin (e.g., shingles) to the ribcage (e.g., costochondritis), pleura (e.g., mesothelioma), lungs (e.g., pneumonia, pulmonary infarct, mass-forming lesion such as cancer), heart layers (e.g., pericarditis, myocardial infarction), great vessels (e.g., pulmonary embolism), and finally the esophagus (e.g., esophageal rupture). This mental exercise aids memory consolidation of human anatomy but also facilitates a systematic analysis of potential causes that could account for a patient presentation.

Overlaying this anatomical approach with the **VITAMIN CDE mnemonic** enhances diagnostic precision by incorporating etiological categories into the anatomical framework. For instance, within the lung as an anatomical structure, vascular causes might include pulmonary embolism; infectious causes could be pneumonia; neoplastic causes might be primary lung carcinoma or metastases; and autoimmune causes could include sarcoidosis. Integrating these two approaches makes a thorough exploration of both systemic and localized disease processes much easier to construct.

However, context is always the key to narrowing down differentials effectively. The clinical history and physical exam, results from any imaging the patient went through, blood or laboratory results, and any other clues must guide this process—otherwise, you risk overburdening yourself with an exhaustive list of possibilities for every patient, offering little practical value. The merging of anatomical localization and etiological categorization described above provides a structured but flexible method for creating effective differential diagnoses across all medical specialties. These frameworks are important tools in navigating the intricate web of potential diagnoses that might account for patient presentations in daily medical practice, regardless of specialty.

Suggested Readings

1. Longacre TA. Mills and Sternberg's diagnostic surgical pathology. 7th ed. Wolters Kluwer Health; 2021.
2. Nature reviews disease primers [Internet]. London: Springer Nature Limited; 2026 [cited 2026 Feb 11]. https://www.nature.com/nrdp/
3. UMass Chan Medical School, Center for Academic Achievement. Strategies for generating differential diagnoses [Internet]. Worcester (MA): UMass Chan Medical School; 2006 [cited 2026 Feb 11]. https://www.umassmed.edu/globalassets/clinical-faculty-development-center/nov-2017-w1t1-materials/10e-differential-dx-strategies---online.pdf

5 Cellular Rebellion

The human body can be conceptualized as a cellular metropolis, where millions of residing cells interact in a dynamic harmony to maintain health and enable effective and smooth bodily functions. Within this environment, however, a coup can arise without a moment's notice. This bustling city is full of microscopically small citizens (the cells) performing tasks and jobs that are integral to the community at large: muscle cells contract to allow us to move or to move food through the gut, neurons transmit signals to enable sensation and perception, and immune cells patrol or wait for invaders to maintain this peace. Their collective efforts under normal conditions establish an equilibrium, upholding the general health of each and every one of us. In this bodily kingdom, a realm ruled by unyielding biophysical laws, it takes only one subject to abjure the natural order and repurpose these protocols for conquest. These aforementioned biophysical laws represent the fundamental processes that govern cellular life: the precise replication of DNA and coordinated division of cells, strictly programmed cell death (apoptosis), maintenance of electrical and chemical gradients to allow proper cellular functioning, among others. Each law ensures that cells act not for selfish gain but in concert with their neighbours, adhering to tightly regulated schedules and behaviours—directly analogous to the provisions and processes that keep a city running smoothly.

N. Pardell, *Scalpel, Scope, and Stain*,
https://doi.org/10.1007/978-3-032-25384-2_5

A single cell that goes rogue, initiated by a genetic mutation or other molecular aberration, breaches its code of conduct—igniting an insurgency. A genetic mutation is an error in the DNA sequence of a cell, which can be either inherited at the time of conception or acquired from the environment through exposure to radiation or toxins or even just from mistakes during DNA replication in the cell. While many mutations are repaired or result in no significant consequences, some mutations strike at just the right location to disrupt the genetic script controlling the growth and even behaviour of the cell. This breach of protocol is akin to a law-abiding citizen suddenly becoming a rebel leader, ignoring authoritative rules to focus on personal ambitions. The rogue cell's descendants, inheriting the initial mutations of its ancestor (and therefore ambitious drive), multiply and divide with reckless abandon and carve out territories in tissues never meant to host such anarchy. These progeny—the direct descendants of the original rogue cell—acquire not only the same genetic errors but, in time, may pick up additional mutations, each one potentially bestowing new survival advantages much like a neophyte criminal syndicate arming itself with unconventional tools or unorthodox tactics.

Soon, they diverge into disparate factions, each employing new strategies to secure control of the local and global—once peaceful—ecosystem. Some cells hack into the blood vessel routes, transporting themselves to distant, distinct habitats; others camouflage themselves to evade immune sentinels. This diversity among cell populations within the same tumour is known in scientific terms as tumour heterogeneity—a hallmark of established cancers where different 'subclones' or subpopulations develop within a single tumour mass. Each subclone carries specific genetic changes, called subclonal mutations, in addition to the ancestral mutations conferred from the original rogue leader's mission. These subclones—each armed with unique genetic blueprints but all equipped with the original mutations of the original rogue cell—compete in a Darwinian-style arena, where only the most ruthless survive. This Darwinian arena refers to the evolutionary pressures that exist inside the tumour: cells that grow faster, hide better from immunity, or resist therapy will outlast and outnumber weaker competitors, selecting for and propelling the tumour's evolution just as predator-prey dynamics and natural selection shape populations in the wild. Like rival dynasties vying for a throne, they adapt and undergo selection, acquiring functions and powers their ancestors never possessed. The tumour becomes a mosaic of microdomains, its variation a living testament to evolution's perpetual experimentation. It is this ever-shifting landscape of cell populations—constantly mutating, adapting, and evolving new survival mechanisms—that makes treating cancer so challenging, as no two areas of a tumour may be exactly alike, and new clones can emerge in response to therapy (a major selection pressure among cancer).

Mutations arise at random—some fortifying the sect, others leading to their ruin—and the milieu shifts with each cellular generation. Genetic changes can be neutral, beneficial, or even detrimental to a cancer clone. The fate of any given mutation is determined by its effect on survival and proliferation within the shifting local context—be it exposure to chemotherapy, a particularly vigilant immune response, or the availability of vital nutrients. Some new clones may go extinct quite rapidly, while others thrive due to the advantages they have gained, reshaping the cancer's behaviour. The result is ongoing, branching evolution within a single person: a process far more chaotic than any predictable, linear model. What begins as a monolithic revolt soon fragments into myriad clandestine battlefields, where yesterday's ally becomes today's adversary. It is not uncommon for subclones within one tumour to compete directly for scarce resources, or even temporarily form an allegiance to outperform stronger rivals, reminiscent of both competition and uneasy alliances familiar from political or military spheres. The pathologist, peering into this tumultuous canvas, faces not a uniform enemy but a transforming legion, frozen in time on a glass slide—a survival story reminiscent of Darwin's sketches, but unfolding at a breakneck pace.

Microscopic examination reveals this drama via regions of distinct cellular appearances, patterns of cell death, and the emergence of odd, hybrid visual appearances, also known as morphologies—a visible record of evolutionary struggle that is often only partially captured in a single slide or biopsy. Here, in the microcosm of a slide, lies the paradox of cancer: a disease born of self, yet alien in its ambition. Every cell that wages this war was derived from the patient's own genetic material, yet has become unrecognizable—following rules and pursuing goals entirely its own. This dual nature underlies the tragic, transformative, and terrifying aspects of malignancy—self against self, order collapsing into chaos. To diagnose the process is to decode a living and dynamic fossil record—one where every nucleus and stain applied to it whispers tales of adaptation, betrayal, and the fragile line between balance and discord. Much as paleontologists interpret the fossil record for clues to the ancient past, so too do pathologists interpret cellular morphology and arrangement as evidence for the 'history' of each tumour, reconstructing its rise from a single aberrant cell to a world unto itself. Unlike the fossil record, which unfolded over millennia, cancer's evolution plays out in months, weeks, and sometimes even days. Tumour evolution is measured not in epochs but in clinical time; a malignancy can fundamentally change its character over a chemotherapy cycle, rapidly spawning new traits and vulnerabilities—or resistance. Thus, treatment is sometimes a race against this micro-evolutionary clock. The pathologist often sits at the veil between the world seen with the naked eye and the world at war through the microscope. To the surgeon, a tumour may appear consistent, but under the microscope, the battle lines and shifting territory are evident. The pathologist, decoding these patterns, becomes translator, historian, and strategist—bridging the seen and unseen worlds of cancer.

Cancer is not one disease but thousands of distinct diseases and is a topic that pathologists must know extremely well. The term 'cancer' is, in reality, an umbrella encompassing a vast spectrum of conditions, each defined by specific genetic mutations, tissue origins, biological behaviours, response patterns to therapies, and clinical impact. Modern oncology recognizes that even within a single organ, cancers can diverge dramatically in how they look under the microscope, what mutations drive their growth, their likelihood for recurrence after treatment, or their propensity to metastasize. In fact, most surgical pathologists see cancer every day, in various organs, and in various forms. Through analyzing the cancerous combatants individually, their architecture and battle formations as a group, and the battlefield itself, including the normal adjacent tissues and the immune system counter-offensive, the pathologist makes poignant observations and critical determinations. Such observations include the type of cancer seen, if it arose in the location the clinical team found it in, or it travelled from a not-yet-discovered site in the patient, and how far along the cancer is in its annexation of normal tissues. For example, determining whether a lung mass is a primary lung cancer or a metastasis from a different organ profoundly affects prognosis and dictates the patient's treatment plan. Staging, such as how far the tumour has invaded neighbouring organs or lymph nodes, is likewise essential for guiding therapy. Through various quantitative and qualitative methods, the pathologist drafts a report conveying the salient features of the cancer resected by the surgeon, replete with all of the information that has been proven clinically significant to portend prognostic and therapeutic insights. This includes details such as tumour grade, stage, the presence of lymphatic or vascular vessel invasion, the status of margins, and the results of immunohistochemical or molecular studies—each metric contributing to a nuanced clinical picture for the treating team.

The cell is the basic unit of life, and most can undergo division and propagate their traits to their descendants. Cells can move in response to stimuli and signals from the environment and sense the presence of other cells. Cells can produce their own substances and molecules. They can protect, regulate, process, absorb, and/or secrete. As you can imagine, the interconnectedness of these responses forms a highly complex system, where various simultaneous signals are integrated by the cell through numerous cellular 'pathways' involving a multitude of proteins. Each cell in the body is constantly receiving, processing, and reacting to a plethora of internal and external cues. These can include hormones, growth factors, signals from neighbouring cells, and feedback from the extracellular matrix—the complex scaffolding that supports cells and transmits information. The regulated orchestration of these pathways is what maintains normal tissue architecture and function.

In its most basic conceptualization, cancer is a pathology that originates from aberrations in an individual cell's genome that lead to unregulated growth and survival of the cell. Since the genome is responsible for providing the blueprint upon which various proteins are created, mutations of various forms may result in altered levels of key proteins, or even altered proteins themselves, and can result in an imbalance between growth-promoting responses to signals, versus growth inhibiting (or death-promoting) responses. This can happen in various ways—perhaps a protein that usually tells the cell to stop dividing becomes inactivated, creating a double negative and, just as two negatives equal a positive in basic arithmetic, promote cell proliferation. Alternatively, a protein that periodically tells the cell to accelerate through the cell cycle (the process by which cells divide into daughter cells) might be altered to be constitutively in the 'on' state, like a car with the accelerator stuck to the floor. Other critical proteins, such as those that repair DNA damage (e.g., BRCA1/2), may cease functioning, allowing the accumulation of mutations at an accelerated rate. These mutations or genetic errors compound over time, giving rise to greater genomic instability and expediting the transformation from a normal cell to a malignant one. The normal 'checkpoints' for cell division and survival that have been implemented by evolution are circumvented through these genetic mutations and altered proteins, resulting in an unstable system and, in the case of cancer, promote its proliferation and expansion into surrounding areas and distant sites it was never intended to inhabit. Without these brakes and checks, the cell—and its descendants—break free of their growth restraints, ignore signals to die, and eventually invade locally, enter blood or lymph vessels, and establish colonies at new bodily sites (metastasize).

Through progressive mutations, cancer can acquire various functions that enable it to act lawlessly. Although there are a staggering number of ways in which these functions can become manifest, the features that define cancer can be grouped into distinct categories known as the *Hallmarks of Cancer*. First outlined by Hanahan and Weinberg in 2000 and refined in 2011, the hallmarks denote fundamental traits exhibited by most cancers. Although such traits can come about from myriad molecular pathways and interactions, specific to different cancer types, the endpoints are largely similar. Such hallmarks include:

1. **Sustaining proliferative signalling**: Cancer cells might generate their own signals to grow or repurpose normal signalling pathways to drive unchecked cell division.

2. **Evading growth suppressors**: Tumours bypass the normal mechanisms that normally limit or halt cell division, through effects on what is known as the 'cell cycle.' One protein that acts (in normal conditions) to moderate cell division in normal tissues includes *p53*, which is the most commonly mutated protein in human cancers.
3. **Resisting cell death**: Cancerous cells avoid a form of cell death known as *apoptosis* by increasing levels of death-inhibiting proteins or disrupting the molecular pathway that drives cell death so that such signals never meet their destinations.
4. **Enabling replicative immortality**: Cancer cells might activate a specific enzyme called *telomerase* or influence alternative chromosome lengthening mechanisms to overcome common limitations in the number of replications they may undergo (known as replicative senescence).
5. **Inducing angiogenesis**: Tumours can secrete proteins such as *VEGF* or other factors to recruit blood vessels for nutrient and oxygen supply, as even cancer cells need oxygen to fuel their behaviours.
6. **Activating invasion and metastasis**: Cancers known as carcinomas acquire motility through a process known as *epithelial-mesenchymal transition* and modify the extracellular matrix (the surrounding network in between cells) to gain access to domains hitherto forbidden.
7. **Reprogramming energy metabolism**: The *Warburg effect* allows cancer cells to prioritize the production of nucleotides, amino acids, and lipids over maximal efficiency in ATP synthesis (ATP being the molecule that is used to power the cell) via a process called aerobic glycolysis.
8. **Evading immune destruction**: Tumours can escape detection by the immune system by increasing expression of a protein known as **PD-L1** to inactivate T-cells, reducing MHC I levels to limit antigen presentation, and attracting regulatory T-cells that actively suppress immune responses.

These hallmarks confer malignant tumours the ability to grow with excessive speed, to spread far and wide, to resist therapeutic agents we throw at them, and to ultimately cause harm to the patient.

The pathologist must remain vigilant for signs of these hallmarks, both morphologically and via special stains and tests, as these clues can help classify disease and inform treatment options.

Not all tumours are cancerous, however. Many neoplasms (meaning 'new growths') are benign, meaning that they remain localized to their site of origin and do not metastasize, or travel to distant sites. Benign tumours are still an issue of growth signalling, albeit more controlled than that of their malignant counterparts. Benign tumours tend to grow slowly, are often well delineated from the surrounding normal tissues, and do not usually show invasion into the surroundings (destruction of the adjacent normal tissue). Although not cancer, such neoplasms can still result in complications and morbidity (and even death) usually by virtue of their size, compressive effects on surrounding structures, and their physiological functions. For example, leiomyomas of the uterus (also known as 'fibroids') are tumours that are derived from the smooth muscle cells of the myometrium, in the wall of the uterus. Although not cancerous, they can result in major complications such as heavy bleeding, sometimes necessitating IV blood transfusions, pelvic pain, constipation (by compressing the rectum), urinary issues (by compressing the bladder), and infertility or pregnancy complications. Large arterial-venous malformations in the brain or liver of neonates can result in a significant low-resistance shunt of blood volume that the newborn goes into high-output congestive heart failure. Pituitary neuroendocrine tumours (benign tumours of the pituitary gland at the base of the brain) can grow so large that they compress the optic chiasm above it, the tract carrying visual information from the retina of the eyes to the back of the brain to be processed. This can result in blindness and headaches. As well, some of these tumours still secrete hormones like the original normal cell they were derived from, leading to endocrinopathies such as acromegaly and Cushing's disease. Benign bone tumours can cause pain, swelling, and fractures.

Malignant tumours, by contrast, are those that embody the hallmarks of cancer, and the most definitive marker of malignancy is metastasis. Malignant tumours are usually faster growing, and often invade surrounding tissues like tendrils of ivy, slithering forth and inserting themselves between normal tissue such that their boundaries are often ill-defined. Their destructive capability, and the ability for the malignancy to travel to distant sites of the body like the lungs, brain, bone, and liver and continue its incessant goals of expansion are what make cancer distinct from benign neoplasms.

A lung cancer arising at the apex of the lung provides a masterclass in the consequences of unchecked cellular invasion. These so-called Pancoast tumours, most often *non-small cell lung carcinomas*, are uniquely positioned to encroach upon the neurovascular crossroads of the thoracic inlet. As the tumour expands, it can invade or compress the T1 nerve root and the preganglionic sympathetic fibres as they ascend toward the stellate ganglion—an anatomical relay station nestled at the junction of the cervical and thoracic sympathetic chains. This disruption in the neuronal circuit known as the 'oculosympathetic' pathway halts the signals responsible for pupillary dilation and upper eyelid elevation, culminating in the clinical constellation of Horner's syndrome. The result is unmistakable: ipsilateral ptosis from denervation of Müller's muscle, miosis due to unopposed parasympathetic tone, and anhidrosis from loss of sympathetic innervation to the facial sweat glands. The face on the affected side betrays the tumour's silent progression—an eyelid that droops, a pupil that refuses to dilate, and skin that grows dry and pale. Far from a mere neurological curiosity, Horner's syndrome in this context is a signpost of local tumour aggression, its presence a testament to the intimate relationship between anatomy and disease.

As I described in an earlier chapter, when seeing the *morphology* of the tumour at hand, a differential diagnosis is generated. Once I have decided that the process I am seeing under the microscope is in fact neoplastic (versus inflammatory, infectious, etc.), I then try to determine if it is benign versus malignant. Various features help in this distinction, and some are more helpful in specific cancer types than others. Commonly, cancer cells show large, dark nuclei with irregular borders. There might be a large nucleolus. The cells might be pleomorphic, meaning that relative to other cancer cells, they vary in size and shape. Architecturally, the tumour may be ill-defined, and I cannot draw a nice circle around the growing mass to delineate its boundaries precisely. They may have evidence of necrosis (unregulated cell death), often due to outgrowing its blood supply and dying due to lack of oxygen.

Another clue to malignancy under the microscope is that numerous and even atypical mitotic figures can be seen. As a cell divides, it must go through mitosis, a process of cell division where the chromosomes condense, aggregate at a cellular equator, and are partitioned into two domains before the cytoplasm pinches off and produces two independent cells. We can see this process under the microscope, and it serves as a marker of how fast the neoplasm is growing. The more proliferative, usually the more likely it is malignant.

Once we decide a tumour is malignant, we must now decide what type of cancer it is, usually by figuring out what kind of cell the cancer arose from, or put another way, its **line of differentiation**. Broadly, a cancer can be a **carcinoma**, a **sarcoma**, a **hematopoietic** neoplasm (such as a lymphoma), a **germ cell** neoplasm, a **glial** neoplasm, a **neuroendocrine** neoplasm, and, never forget, a **melanoma**.

Different cells, by virtue of their location, biological activity and roles, have different proteins and other biomolecules they express, different intracellular infrastructure, and different pathways they rely on. If a malignancy looks very similar to its normal counterpart, it is quite easy to tell what line of differentiation it exhibits just by looking at a simple H&E-stained slide (hematoxylin and eosin is the workhorse stain of pathology used every day). Smooth muscle cells look different from lymphocytes, which look different from squamous cells (such as those that make up the epidermis of the skin). However, sometimes the cancer can look so far removed from the originating cell's appearance that H&E stains cannot be relied on alone. Here we turn to specific ancillary tests and stains to help pick out aspects of the tumour cells that might betray their true lineage. One such technique is known as **immunohistochemistry**.

Immunohistochemistry, or IHC for short, is the pathologist's secret codebreaker device—a technique that lets us unmask the identity of cells hiding in plain sight. When faced with a tumour that refuses to declare its lineage (also known as a poorly differentiated tumour), we turn to antibodies: specialized proteins that can be crafted to seek out and attach to unique molecular 'badges,' known as antigens, worn by different cell types. Almost anything in a cell can be considered an antigen if it can be detected by this mechanism. Imagine an antigen as an identification badge and the antibody we apply to the glass slide as a scanner—if the badge is present in that cell, the scanner detects it, painting the cell brown and those without it remaining a blank canvas (which appears blue). With discerning eyes, we can analyze the chromatic patterns that develop as a result of this technique to ultimately determine if the cells we actually wanted to interrogate are 'positive' for that antibody (are stained brown).

But the story seldom ends with the unmasking of just one antigen. No antibody is a perfect detective—many cell types share antigens, and the same marker can appear in unexpected places. Take Thyroid Transcription Factor 1 (TTF-1): Using an antibody to TTF-1 results in a positive signal in most lung and thyroid tumours but can also be positive in tumours of the endometrium or those known as 'neuroendocrine' tumours. A brown-stained nucleus tells us we're on our way, but usually not at the finish line yet. The art of using this technique in pathology lies in the integration of multiple clues: starting with the patterns we see on the trusty H&E stain, then issuing a tailored *panel* of antibodies to different antigens to narrow the differential diagnostic playing field. Only through the combination of morphology, clinical context, and a judicious selection of antibodies do we reveal the tumour's true nature, avoiding the pitfalls of false certainty. In this way, IHC is not just a test—it's a dance between science and intuition, an interplay that leads us to the truth about the tumour, one stain at a time. In addition to traditional histology and immunohistochemistry, modern pathology increasingly relies on molecular diagnostics—techniques such as next-generation sequencing (NGS), fluorescence in situ hybridization (FISH), and polymerase chain reaction (PCR)—to detect genetic mutations, chromosomal alterations, and other molecular abnormalities that drive tumour behaviour. These powerful tools not only refine our ability to classify cancers but also guide targeted therapies and personalized treatment decisions.

Cancer is a formidable adversary, ever-changing through mutations and epigenetic alterations, adapting under the selective pressures of chemotherapy and immune surveillance. As discussed above, the biology of cancer is not homogeneous, and subtle clues are engraved in the architecture and appearance of cells—clues that may betray its future course in the patient. In this landscape, the pathologist stands as both chronicler and scryer: a chronicler, meticulously recording the tumour's past and present in the language of morphology and molecular markers; and a scryer, tasked with divining the arcane patterns beneath the microscope into prognostic and actionable insights for clinicians. Pathologists attempt to derive order from the chaotic and kaleidoscopic milieu of tumour cells and subpopulations that arise from the Darwinian crucible, striving to extract absolutes and definitive classifications from an entity inexorably marching toward entropy.

This cellular rebellion is not waged on a static field—it is a chess match where the rules and pieces shift with every moment of time. The hallmarks of cancer—unchecked growth, evasion of death, invasion, and more—are its tactical manoeuvres, deployed in response to the body's defenses and our therapeutic interventions. The relentless diversity of these insurgent cells breeds diagnostic uncertainty, especially in rare tumours, those with ambiguous morphology, or antigenic signatures that defy expectation. Pathology is thus a discipline of shades of grey, not of black-and-white certainty often assumed. A key part of our role is to communicate this uncertainty to clinicians, offering the best possible guidance in the moment, while acknowledging the limits imposed by the ever-evolving nature of the disease. In so doing, we maximize the benefit for the patient, seeking to quell the rebellious and insurgent cells and restore a measure of order to the cellular ecosystem. In the grand contest between chaos and control, the pathologist's lens becomes both the historian's pen and the strategist's compass—bearing witness to the rebellion and shaping the response.

Suggested Readings

1. Hanahan D, Weinberg RA. Hallmarks of cancer: the next generation. Cell. 2011;144(5):646–74.
2. Kumar V, Abbas AK, Aster JC, Debnath J, Das A. Robbins, Cotran & Kumar pathologic basis of disease. 11th ed. Philadelphia: Elsevier; 2025.
3. Weinberg RA. The biology of cancer. 3rd ed. New York (NY): W. W. Norton & Company; 2023.

6 The Silent Teachers

When it comes to medical education for a health professional, there are many avenues to impart knowledge to a keen and engaged student. From practical hands-on experiences on the wards, didactic lectures, informal 'pimping' on the wards (where a senior resident or attending physician quiz learners in a public forum to the point of failure), to self-study; the learning seems endless. The old adage that medical education is like 'drinking water from a fire hose' rings true, and it can be daunting to expect to accumulate the sea of knowledge that always seems to be growing faster than the pace at which you can retain it. But no form of teaching is as enigmatic, visceral and impactful as that which is extended to pathology residents from mentors who have departed the corporeal world. Learning from these silent teachers in the form of autopsy examinations can be a surreal experience, especially in the early stages of training. The benefits to medical education and to the virtues of compassion and respect that can not only be learned, but felt, are tantamount to the development of competent, moral, and discerning pathologists.

The history of the autopsy is a fascinating subject that reflects the evolution of medical science and innovations in the understanding of human anatomy and disease processes. Many sources can be sought that elucidate this rich history, where one would learn about famous figures in medicine such as Andreas Vesalius, Giovanni Morgagni, Karl von Rokitansky, and Rudolf Virchow, as well as

N. Pardell, *Scalpel, Scope, and Stain*,
https://doi.org/10.1007/978-3-032-25384-2_6

their contributions to advancing medicine and pathology. In fact, many of the methods used in modern-day autopsies are largely the same or modified versions of those employed by these prominent figures. Such methods include the order and manner in which organs are procured from bodies or dissected to obtain relevant information as to the disease process, cause of death of the individual, for public health surveillance of disease incidence, and for quality assurance for clinicians and surgeons as to the effectiveness (or ineffectiveness) of particular interventions performed upon the patient while alive.

In doing an autopsy, a pathology resident gains the opportunity to directly witness the effect of medical and surgical disease on the body, both anatomically and functionally. In this manner, a thorough understanding of *pathophysiology* is attained, as direct observation of the changes in organ structure and function finally transcends that learned solely from rote study or microscopic examination. It is this *clinical-pathological* correlation that solidifies and makes tangible the information gleaned from the textbook, cementing one's learning.

The word 'morgue' often provokes visions of an austere, cold, and foreboding place, relegated to the basement away from prying eyes, shimmering with stainless steel counters, lockers, and procedure tables. To a degree, this is accurate—stainless steel affords an easy-to-clean surface after all. However, during an autopsy, it is not uncommon to have the radio playing top 40's hits, like surgeons do in the operating room, with bright lights and some company, whether it be residents like me or pathologists' assistants helping with the dissections. Although still located in the basement at my home institution, it was far from the dreary and foreboding schematic my mind drafted up when first thinking about pathology and autopsies. Now it is a place of respect, learning, and discovery. However, autopsies can come with their own set of emotional challenges, especially as they pertains to pediatrics.

Children should not die, nor suffer the burden or morbidity of disease, especially that resulting from cancer, as the treatment protocols themselves can cause an abundance of side effects, all without a true guarantee of cure. However, intellectually speaking, children and adolescent are subject to the same laws of physics that adults are, down to the elementary level. They have immune systems, some still developing, that sometimes falter, leading to infections such as *C. difficile* colitis and autoimmune diseases such as Crohn's disease. They can suffer from mutations of their DNA within a subset of cells, either present at the beginning of fertilization, throughout embryogenesis, or after birth, which causes an increase in proteins causing unregulated cellular growth and division. As we have seen, this is one mechanism in which cancer arises in general, as cancer is a disease of aberrant genetic blueprints within cells allowing the cells to grow with reckless abandon and to even gain functions that their cell type normally would not have. Other times, the genetic or epigenetic changes result in a loss of a protein in the cell that acts to suppress growth and promote cell death. The result is the same, except the cell growth and division are a result of a lack of brakes (like a runaway train).

This intellectual analysis must be kept in check, however, to ensure the maintenance of the more human aspects of medicine, such as compassion and empathy. Taking a moment to feel for the patient in front of you or to try and imagine the pain and burden on the caregivers can help one maintain their humanity in medicine, where most of what you see is disease, morbidity, and loss. It is a delicate balance, however, as the skill to distance oneself appropriately from the vagaries of the patient's experience is immensely useful and necessary to truly help them. I believe this to be true in all specialties of medicine, and I believe autopsies can be approached similarly.

One day I was in the resident room at another institution during an elective rotation, doing my daily duties reading patient charts and drafting reports that I would review with my assigned staff pathologist for the rotation. I was also on the autopsy service, and any autopsy that came to the hospital would go through me. I received an email regarding an upcoming autopsy—a pediatric autopsy—that I would be involved in. Upon reading that the patient was a newborn baby, I had to stop what I was doing and process. This would be my first pediatric autopsy, an examination that differs from adult autopsies in many ways. I was way out of my league here but thankfully and rightfully so, the pediatric pathologist on service would spearhead the case with my assistance. I did not know how I would feel seeing a baby on those stainless-steel tables, let alone know how I would react or feel to what was surely to be a surreal experience.

I felt for the family, and for the child, and had to prepare myself mentally to undergo the procedure.

The baby had an antenatally diagnosed heart defect, a congenital (present at birth) anomaly. For example, one such defect (among many) seen in premature infants is aortic stenosis—when the aortic valve at the beginning of the large tube that carries oxygen-laden blood to the body's tissues (the aorta) is drastically narrowed, resulting in the heart upstream of the narrowing having to adapt to the situation by working extra hard to pump the same amount of blood to the body as in the normal state to keep everything running smoothly. This is known as *cardiac output*, or the amount of blood exiting the heart chamber through the aorta in each heartbeat. The adaptations the heart undergoes to maintain cardiac output in this setting take a toll, however, and after a brief time this adaptation decompensates, resulting in lower cardiac output and thereby less oxygen going to the body. The patient then starts to deteriorate clinically, showing symptoms of this lack of oxygen. Due to similar symptoms from this particular patient's congenital anomaly, the cardiac surgery service had to operate on the child. Despite the operation, the patient continued to deteriorate due to continued low cardiac output and the sequelae of shock, and further highly specialized medical therapies and optimization had to be implemented.

Despite further imaging studies and tests and optimizing therapies, the medical team could not get the child's cardiorespiratory function to perform adequately. After extensive discussion with the clinical team, the parents opted to remove life-sustaining therapy. The child then passed away.

The autopsy was surreal from the moment I laid eyes on the baby. He was bundled up, lying in a bassinet. I will not delve into the intricacies of this case's examination here, but I will illustrate the role the autopsy had in helping the clinical team understand the child's deterioration and inability to optimize their organ functioning.

Without any specific details, there were significant abnormalities in the patient's cardiovascular system. Ultimately, the findings corroborated the fact that the medical interventions performed were unable to stabilize the patient, due to patient-specific factors that could not have been known in the moment. The possibility was also raised that due to the invasive procedure, an ischemic event may have compounded upon the patient's already precarious cardiac function (a known unavoidable complication for invasive procedures). As a result, the patient was unable to get adequately oxygenated blood from the lungs to their tissues, resulting in decompensation.

Such a case provides the needed closure for the family and provides insight into the efficacy of prior medical interventions for quality assurance purposes. This case also illustrates the valuable feedback loop that autopsy can provide for the medical team, and helps educate those involved in a patient's care as to the scenarios that may occur. Such a case also demands the human side of the pathologist. It is not easy to perform a pediatric autopsy, both technically and emotionally. But it is a vital and necessary job to provide much-needed answers, especially for the family.

Another case I had was of an adult male with a remote history of construction work. He presented with a 1-month history of increasing pedal edema (swelling of the legs), abdominal distension and shortness of breath. His past medical history was notable for COPD (a chronic lung disease), gastroesophageal reflux disease, and hypertension (high blood pressure). Upon opening the chest, everything appeared quite normal. Upon opening the abdominal cavity, however, the answers declared themselves. The abdominal cavity was coated throughout with pungent-smelling, white and red thick masses and plaques that made the abdominal organs adhere to each other and to the abdominal wall. The whole mesentery (the fatty and vascular tissue that routes blood from the aorta to the abdominal organs) was also infiltrated by massive amounts of the material. In addition, there was an exuberant amount of white pus and fluid that had collected in the abdomen. After a lengthy extraction of the organs, as they were all adherent and hidden in the sea of disease, sections were taken to determine microscopically what these masses were composed of and to understand the extent of the disease.

Under the microscope it was apparent that we were dealing with a *mesothelioma*, a cancer of the lining of the body cavities. Usually, mesothelioma occurs in the pleural cavity lining the lungs or chest wall. It is much less common having a mesothelioma that arises from the lining of the abdominal cavity, as seen in this case. This discrepancy is due in part to the exposure of the pleural cavity and lungs to environmental and often occupational carcinogens inhaled by the patient. With the patient's history of construction work when asbestos was ubiquitous, asbestosis was high up on the differential for causing such a cancer. Despite being in the abdominal cavity, it has been documented that asbestos is a risk factor for abdominal primary mesothelioma as well, albeit much more rarely than the pleural counterpart. On the microscopic sections, we performed Perl's Prussian Blue special stain, which highlights the element iron, allowing us to see the iron-containing proteins adsorbed onto the asbestos material that does not degrade to confirm the presence of occupationally acquired asbestos deposition in the body. This case had implications for the family as it relates to the Worker's Compensation Board, allowing them to receive compensation due to the intimate causation between mesothelioma and occupational exposure to asbestos.

The last case I wanted to share is a case of a man who presented to the emergency department with nonspecific chest pain. The emergency doctors did a thorough workup for ischemic heart disease and other pathologies without finding a particular cause for his recurring chest pain. He developed a cardiac tamponade a little while later (where fluid or blood collects in the pericardial cavity and, due to being quite indistensible, compresses the heart and reduces cardiac output). The patient underwent an emergency pericardiectomy, where the cardiac surgeons opened this space to drain the fluid and relieve the tamponade of the heart. However, the patient eventually went into cardiac arrest and passed away. It remained unclear as to the origin of his chest pain and eventual cardiac arrest, let alone the pericardial effusion.

During the external examination at autopsy, the patient had lots of evidence of medical intervention (IV's, EKG leads, drains, etc.). On examination of the heart, I noticed a large blood clot on the surface that, on removal, revealed a very large *hole* in the heart. This patient died due to ventricular rupture post-myocardial infarction (a 'heart attack'). This means that high-pressure blood blew through the wall of the heart. Microscopically, we could date the time of the heart attack as approximately 1 week prior to death. Interestingly, due to the necrotic tissue and the subsequent inflammation and remodelling of heart muscle after a myocardial infarct, the structural integrity of the wall is weakest from around the 3–7 day mark, because there is time for neutrophils and macrophages to 'clean up' the debris, but not enough time for the fibroblasts to lay down enough collagen to result in thick scar tissue. Ventricular wall rupture is a known complication after a heart attack, and ultimately led to this patient's death. Thus, this patient had a prior heart attack causing chest pain that evaded detection (no test in medicine is 100% sensitive and specific), resulting in death via a complication (rupture through the thinned wall of the damaged heart tissue) thereof around 1 week later.

As you can see, autopsies offer technical, medical, and emotional information to those who conduct them and to those who were involved in the patient's care. These 'silent teachers' offer an educational opportunity for residents and staff pathologists that go beyond that of the textbook or lecture slide. With direct visualization and handling of pathology directly, the pathologist is able to consolidate their understanding of disease with the patient's story, blending humanity and scientific rigour. The empathy and respect afforded by autopsy to trainees is an overlooked benefit of this practice, as it helps one remain grounded and even provides a springboard for one to contemplate one's own mortality. In the end, these silent teachers leave an indelible mark on those who listen closely, guiding them to become not just skilled diagnosticians but also thoughtful stewards of patient care.

Suggested Readings

1. Burton JL, Underwood JCE. Clinical, educational, and epidemiological value of autopsy. Lancet. 2007;369(9571):1471–1480.
2. Hooper JE, Williamson AK, editors. Autopsy in the 21st century: best practices and future directions [Internet]. Cham: Springer; 2019 [cited 2026 Feb 11]. https://doi.org/10.1007/978-3-319-98373-8.

7 Frozen Under the Knife

Pathology, due to the rate-limiting step of specimen processing time by the laboratory, often proceeds at a steady pace, immune to external pressures to produce results. Tissue needs to be fixed for a specific duration of time, or else analysis and diagnosis are compromised. One of my preceptors once told me that when a surgeon called for a diagnosis of a tumour they resected the day before, she told him 'would you like the quick answer, or the correct one?' He promptly submitted to the latter and hung up the phone. There are instances where a case can be marked 'STAT' so as to prioritize these specimens for processing, but the fixation time bottleneck still exists.

However, there is a common scenario where a diagnosis must be rendered within 20 min to guide patient management and ensure patient safety. This is known as the 'frozen section.' There are multiple indications for a surgeon to request a frozen section from a pathologist but they all have in common the fact that there is a patient under anesthesia in the operating room in the midst of an operation. The surgeon commonly wants to know the status of *margins* if the patient is there for an oncologic resection (surgical removal of cancer). The surgeon may have resected the tumour so that, to the naked eye, there is none left in the patient. However, as discussed before, cancer is a fickle phenomenon. If there is a cancerous cell left in the patient, the risk of recurrence for that cancer shoots upwards. The surgeon will send the outer aspects of the resection cavity (with

N. Pardell, *Scalpel, Scope, and Stain*,
https://doi.org/10.1007/978-3-032-25384-2_7

a demarcation of *orientation*, such as superior, inferior, etc.) for frozen section analysis.

The specimen is shuttled to the frozen section room, where a pathologist is waiting for it after being paged just moments before that this must be done. The piece of tissue is quickly subject to a gross examination, mounted on a metal slab and coated in a medium that allows quick freezing of the tissue. The tissue is cut into very thin (measured in micrometres) sections in a cryotome and quickly stained according to institutional protocols. Within 20 min and often less, the tissue is looked at under the microscope in the same room, and the pathologist must make some critical determinations.

Analyzing frozen section tissue has its own challenges that conventional 'permanent' sections do not, termed 'artifacts.' For example, the quick freezing often results in cracks in the tissue, altering the architecture seen under the microscope. Fat within the tissue, if present, does not cut well when frozen and can result in large holes in the tissue. Some nuclear atypia (where the cell nuclei do not look 'normal' for their cell type and location) can result from the quick freezing, leading to a dilemma when deciding if the atypical cells and nuclei are a result of malignant transformation or merely the freezing itself. It is these aspects of frozen sections that can produce some anxiety or trepidation and result in some of the more adrenaline-filled moments of a pathologist's career. In the example of margin assessment, seeing cancerous cells (a *positive margin*) during the intraoperative consultation means that some cancer could theoretically be left behind in the patient, necessitating the surgeon to continue with their resection at that location. A *negative margin* is the desired result, where the tissue under the microscope does not harbour malignant cells. In this scenario, the surgeon 'closes' the patient, the operation ceases, and the patient can be taken off anesthesia.

The rapid diagnosis facilitated by frozen section analysis is crucial in minimizing anesthesia time during surgery. By offering real-time information about the nature of a lesion and its extent, frozen sections enable surgeons to make immediate decisions about the extent of surgery needed while the patient remains on the operating table. The surgeon can then make further decisions if required during this operation instead of having the patient undergo follow-up surgeries had they waited 1–2 days for the typical *permanent* sections to be reported. The quick turnaround time afforded by frozen sections also reduces the duration of anesthesia exposure. Minimizing anesthesia time is particularly important as prolonged exposure can lead to various physiological risks, including respiratory complications, cardiovascular issues, thromboembolic complications (e.g., prolonged immobility resulting in a deep vein thrombosis and/or subsequent pulmonary embolus) and increased susceptibility to infections. Therefore, the efficiency of frozen section diagnosis plays a vital role in improving patient safety and surgical outcomes by allowing for prompt and appropriate surgical interventions while keeping anesthesia duration to a minimum.

Sometimes the frozen section is required to delineate the exact diagnosis of a lesion. Other times, it is only to elucidate if *lesional* tissue was extracted, ensuring the surgeon resected the appropriate area containing the lesion. After all, not all lesions are readily discriminated from surrounding normal tissue. For example, in some brain tumours, all that may be seen might be an enlargement of the involved portion of the brain with anatomical landmarks somewhat blending together. Learning the intricacies of frozen section analysis as well as what questions can be asked and answered and those which cannot, is an important part of pathology training and is necessary to provide safe patient care.

On a regular surgical pathology rotation, a common page I might get would be for a frozen section during a thyroidectomy operation. A thyroidectomy is the meticulous surgical removal of the thyroid gland, a bilobed organ situated in the anterior neck in intimate proximity to the trachea. It is a component of the visceral compartment of the neck, along with the trachea, and cervical esophagus. On the posterior aspect, it is in close approximation to the recurrent laryngeal nerves and parathyroid glands, often embedded on the posterior surface or even within the thyroid tissue itself. Laterally are the common carotid arteries, major conduits for blood leaving the heart towards the neck, head, and brain. As one might suspect, thyroidectomy is a delicate procedure for a surgeon to preserve these critical structures. Injury to the recurrent laryngeal nerve can result in hoarseness, as this nerve is responsible for vocal cord movement. Injury to the external branch of the superior laryngeal nerve can lead to an inability to achieve high-pitched sounds and a weakened voice, a voice often described as 'monotonous' or lacking projection, as this nerve controls vocal pitch modulation. Another important structure, especially regarding our discussion on frozen section, is preservation of the parathyroid glands which help regulate calcium metabolism. Inadvertent removal of the parathyroid glands can cause post-operative hypoparathyroidism and resultant hypocalcemia, a serious complication. Parathyroid glands are small, yellow-brown, and due to their complex embryological development and migration, can be found within the substance of the thyroid gland, inferiorly extending into the mediastinum, or even within the thymus gland. Due to their unassuming appearance, they can easily be mistaken for fatty tissue, lymph nodes, thymic tissue, or even thyroid nodules themselves. Surgeons often call for frozen sections during thyroidectomy to confirm that the structure they are seeing is in fact parathyroid or one of these mimics. Frozen section diagnosis of parathyroid tissue helps the surgeon avoid their erroneous removal, especially if the patient has anatomical variations and helps steer the patient away from serious post-operative complications.

Under the microscope, it is often quite easy to tell if the tissue submitted by the surgeon is in fact parathyroid, versus a fat lobule, thymic tissue, thyroid tissue, or a lymph node, as these all have different tissue architecture and cell types. Parathyroids, for example, consist mainly of three distinct cell types—oxyphil, chief, and clear cells. They have a thin capsule and regularly have adipose (fat) tissue embedded within the gland, which increases with age (around 50% replacement by the fifth decade of life).

Some other indications for frozen section, in addition to those noted above, include:

- **Determine the benignity versus malignancy of a mass, influencing the extent of surgery** (e.g., ovarian tumour diagnosed as a serous cystadenoma intraoperatively will lead to a much smaller surgery than a diagnosis of serous carcinoma, where the surgeon may do lymph node dissections and even remove the omentum)
- **Margin assessment during cancer** resection (e.g., in breast-conserving surgery for invasive carcinoma, a positive margin means the surgeon will, in the same operation, remove more tissue,

versus waiting for the permanent sections and bringing the patient back another day)

- **Lymph node evaluation during a cancer staging procedure** (e.g., axillary lymph nodes in breast cancer, where the frozen section results help the surgeon determine if they go on to a complete axillary lymph node dissection or not)
- **Identification of specific tissue types** (e.g., identifying parathyroid glands during thyroidectomy to preserve them and avoid post-operative complications)
- **Confirming lesional tissue** (e.g., Gliomas of the brain may have frozen sections to confirm that the neurosurgeon is targeting the correct area for resection)

When I was on a Neuropathology rotation, we frequently received frozen sections to delineate the diagnostic category of a lesion, directly influencing the extent of resection. For example, if a mass lesion in the brain turns out to be a lymphoma, resection is not indicated, and the surgeon would close the case, and the patient would be afforded systemic treatment. However, if it turns out to be metastatic carcinoma, they will proceed, if safe to do so, with resection. If the lesion was a high-grade glioma, they would go for wide resections to remove as much of the tumour as possible, due to the permeative nature of these cancer cells spreading throughout the brain tissue. In fact, historically, when a glioma was radiologically confined to one lobe or hemisphere of the brain, surgeons such as Walter Dandy have tried to remove the entire involved hemisphere (known as a hemispherectomy) to go for cure. However, this did not lead to a cure, and in addition to the high mortality rates, the tumour inevitably started to regrow on the other side of the brain, due to the diffuse nature of its spread throughout the brain.

Frozen sections operate at the intersection of pathology and surgery, where a rapid diagnostic decision directly impacts a patient's outcome. Although it has its challenges—artifacts due to tissue composition, freezing, and sectioning in the cryostat, as well as time constraints—and sometimes adrenaline-filled moments, frozen section analysis remains indispensable for ensuring safe and precise surgical management. Between confirming margins in an oncologic resection and the identification of critical structures like the parathyroid glands in a thyroidectomy operation, the frozen section process demands the pathologist to demonstrate expertise in navigating uncertainty under pressure and time constraints. These moments are a testament to the collaborative nature of medicine, where pathologists and surgeons work hand-in-hand (or scalpel-to-scalpel) to optimize patient care. As a pathology resident, mastering frozen section analysis is not only a technical skill but also an exercise in adaptability, decision-making, and teamwork—qualities that I have come to know define the essence of this specialty.

Suggested Readings

1. Cipriani NA, Husain AN, Taxy JB. Biopsy interpretation: the frozen section. 3rd ed. Philadelphia: Wolters Kluwer; 2022.
2. Jaafar H. Intra-operative frozen section consultation: concepts, applications and limitations. Malays J Med Sci. 2006;13(1):4–12.

8 The Human Behind the Cells

It is easy in medicine to become so inundated with daily tasks and with the management of the organizational mayhem that inevitably evolves from taking care of a large number of patients that one's emotional and empathetic self can easily be put to the wayside in favor of expediency and necessity. Whether a medical student opts to become a clinician who is patient-facing in the clinic, wards, emergency department, or operating theatre, or whether they decide to become a diagnostician (such as a radiologist or pathologist), they will directly and indirectly impact patient lives through their counsel, diagnoses, and treatments. Akin to Newton's Third Law, it is also a fact that patients and their stories themselves will directly impact the lives of the health practitioners.

During my second year of residency, still trying to understand exactly how to be a pathology resident, I was rotating at a community hospital that often receives gynecologic and breast specimens. I was given a case of a 35-year-old woman who had a routine hysterectomy (removal of the uterus) for abnormal uterine bleeding due to a presumed fibroid (or leiomyoma, in pathologic terms). Imaging showed a large mass within the uterine muscular wall with features suggestive of a large fibroid, a very common benign smooth muscle tumour that can cause symptoms such as abnormal bleeding, pain, and recurrent pregnancy loss. In front of me sat the tray of slides with the standard sections that the pathologists' assistant took from

N. Pardell, *Scalpel, Scope, and Stain*,
https://doi.org/10.1007/978-3-032-25384-2_8

this tumour, a set of representative samples of particular areas of the uterus as well as fallopian tubes. I put the first slide under the microscope, peered into the objective lens, and immediately froze. Despite my limited experience in pathology and especially gynecologic specimens at this time, I could immediately tell that this tumour was not a standard benign fibroid (or leiomyoma). What I saw before me was a very hypercellular mass with cells and nuclei of various shapes and sizes, dark staining nuclei and irregular contours. The cells were arranged in streaming spindled arrays suggestive of smooth muscle lineage (the mass was, after all, arising from the myometrium). Mitotic figures abounded. In general, the tumour looked immediately 'ugly.'

This 35-year-old woman had a leiomyosarcoma, a malignant neoplasm of smooth muscle origin. This was my first oncologic diagnosis that I came to on my own (with verification by multiple attending pathologists much more experienced than me), and I could not help but imagine this woman going home to her kids after her surgery for a 'benign' mass of the uterus, tucking them into bed, satisfied that her bleeding would no longer cause her problems and disrupt her life, unaware of the reality that I was seeing before my eyes. As I was peering at these nefarious cells alone in the resident room, it dawned on me that I was the only person *in the world* who knew that the fate of this woman would now go down a markedly different path than everyone had previously expected. This brought on an uncomfortable, strange sensation within me. I started to imagine the inevitable conversation that the obstetrician-gynecologist would have to have with this woman, and her reaction to realizing she had cancer (especially after hearing the suffix *sarcoma*) the worry involved, and the planning for future follow-up appointments to monitor for recurrence or metastasis. I realized then that pathologists are not immune to the patient experience. It was the first time I felt empathy in pathology transcending the four walls of the room I was situated in, likely due to my direct independent recognition of the malignancy. Every slide is more than a collection of cells frozen in time—it is a snapshot of a person's health, which might have a ripple effect on a multitude of domains in their life. Diagnosing a malignancy can lead to bifurcations in a patient's life trajectory. Side effects from chemotherapy may preclude them from their regular job, impacting their livelihood and financial situation. People can collapse psychologically or inversely realize a hidden robustness within themselves they never knew they had. Physical, emotional, and social factors can all be impacted by a diagnosis, a practice we as pathologists perform every day. The microscope acts as a portal not only to a hidden world of cells and disease, but also as a gate into a patient's life, their resilience, their fears, and their hopes.

On a pediatric pathology elective in the United States, I received a case of an adolescent who was very active, participating in multiple sports and outdoor activities. One day, they were skiing the moguls when they felt a pain deep in their leg. Suspecting an ACL and/or MCL tear, an MRI was performed. The radiology report came back as showing a large destructive lesion located in the metaphysis of their distal femur with periosteal (outer layer of the bone) reaction and significant soft tissue involvement by the mass (stereotypical findings for this entity). The biopsy came back as *osteosarcoma*, a malignant tumour of the bone. However, I did not receive the biopsy and diagnose the osteosarcoma. What I received was an entire leg after amputation. The teenager would go on to receive chemotherapy to try and reduce the risk of metastatic disease, but due to the infiltrative nature of the cancer it was deemed that an above-knee amputation had to be carried out to resect the tumour. The gross examination of such a specimen was otherworldly. It introduced a cognitive dissonance that took time to wrap my head around. Throughout most people's lives, they only associate entire limbs in continuity with a body. Seeing a limb in isolation confused my brain in the beginning, and to this day still stirs a sense of unease within me. Beyond that, I began to think about the patient themselves and their mental well-being—a junior high school student, showing up to school with one leg and on chemotherapy. It takes a special soul to maintain their confidence in the face of the social implications such a surgery would have, especially in such a scholastic setting. Although I did not meet this patient, I understood there would likely be massive implications in their life from such a diagnosis and surgery, and it felt eerie to take a sip of coffee in my comfy chair while projecting into the future the possible outcomes for this patient. The line between detachment and empathic connection is a line known well to most medical practitioners, and in my opinion, the ability to regulate the time and emotional resonance with task-oriented thinking is a skill that is vital in medicine. By moderating the emotional attachment with detachment, one can achieve a balance that preserves the medical practitioner's integrity and emotional capacity and respects the patient's outcomes and burden based on the diagnoses rendered.

This case touched me for another reason as well. I bore witness to Colby Smith, my best friend in high school, an all-star football player and exceptionally intelligent and caring individual get diagnosed with osteosarcoma. In fact, I remember the day he showed symptoms. We were outside during our regular football practice. Colby, an athlete with exceptional endurance who could run fast, for long durations, and with the momentum of a freight train, started to get very short of breath during a routine drill. It became so bad that we had to take his equipment off and let him lie on the ground to catch his breath. Soon after, we could feel the lump along his thoracic spine, protruding outwards. Multiple appointments ensued, a biopsy confirmed osteosarcoma, and his chemotherapy journey began. Throughout this entire process, I never saw Colby shed a single tear. He would give the clothes off his back to help a friend, and never let his diagnosis get in the way of him living his life. His positivity, confidence in a positive outcome, and general happiness were astounding. Later on, he underwent decompressive spinal surgery, but heading into university his health started to decline, but his resolve did not. Despite the medical challenges and emotional toll that must have been present, I would chat with Colby about something cool I learned in physics, and he would tell me about his fascination with the field of sociology after procuring and reading a textbook on the subject. There was never a point in his journey where he wanted attention paid to his diagnosis or challenges. He wrangled every ounce of joy he could from every moment in life, even the small ones. He truly saw a routine drive with a friend as a gift. I truly believe Colby's resolve and determination to see the positives in life even when faced with immense challenges impacted everyone who interacted with him. It has influenced my approach to life—to live fully, to love deeply, and to take risks. We do, after all, have one life, and it sometimes is shorter than one might usually expect. I am forever grateful to Colby for exemplifying what it truly means to be happy with what one has.

Nowhere else is emotional resilience tested than that of the medical examiner's suite. Walking through the morgue on a regular Tuesday, preparing for the eleven forensic autopsy cases that will be performed on rows of stainless steel tables, produces an eerie sensation. All around you, embedded in the clinical histories of the patient bodies who can no longer return your gaze, are unfortunate accidents, intentional demise, and everything in between. Much like the neurosurgical intensive care unit I was exposed to in medical school, you would think that being surrounded by sadness and witnessing patients being victim to life's most tragic deliverances would evoke a depressing atmosphere, the air you breathe leaving a void in your lungs. But it is not the case; the medical examiner's suite was counterintuitively one of the most supportive, lively, and inspiring places I have worked. It is a hub of learning and discovery, a sanctum where questions are posed and answers are directly sought, not solely by the medical examiner, but by an entire team—residents, pathologists' assistants, clinicians, technicians, and students—all acting with a collective mission. Each case is a medical mystery: an opportunity to contemplate pathophysiology, confirm or revise diagnoses, and provide essential closure for families. The medical examiner's suite, in a similar vein to the intensive care unit, is alive with teamwork and camaraderie. Like any bustling critical care unit or emergency room, it relies on the harmony of a diverse team—each person bringing technical, anatomical, forensic, and investigative acumen to the table. The synergistic strengths of each person come together to provide a detailed and complete picture of a patient's story. Knowledge is traded back and forth, jokes float above stainless steel, and playlists—whether rap, indie, or Mozart—fill the air much as they do atop the intensity of an operating theater.

Emotionally, too, the autopsy room resounds with purposeful intent. There is no place for morbid fixation or resignation; it is an environment infused with meaning, where silent teachers continue their vital lessons, bestowing knowledge and wisdom long after life has ended. There is a deep satisfaction in knowing that through our team efforts, we help families find closure and clinicians pursue the highest quality standards of care, often providing definitive explanations for an unexpected loss. The place is rife with feelings of challenge and a sense of urgency. Particularly during complex medico-legal cases, sudden deaths, or teaching sessions, there is a palpable sense of focus—the team's curiosity and mission to answer hard questions fosters a sense of meaning that is, if anything, invigorating rather than enfeebling.

In terms of the physical structure of the modern autopsy suite, this too upends expectation. The suites are bright, impeccably clean, and equipped for safe practice and efficient operations. These rooms are a far cry from popular characterizations to that of basements reminiscent of medieval dungeons. In fact, they are often extremely well illuminated, bathed in the glow of high-powered fluorescent light. As I've reflected elsewhere, it is not uncommon for the air to be awash with musical scores, filling the space with the kind of energy more familiar to an operating theatre than a tomb.

The medical examiner's suite is a place of both technical growth and personal reflection. Each case compels the team of health professionals to deepen their scientific rigor, while also demanding a reverence for the humanity at the core of all medicine. Time and again, these autopsy experiences demand us to process complex emotions, instilling notions of empathy and resilience that we practitioners carry forward—to the benefit of the living, and in honour of those who have passed.

In these ways, the autopsy suite subverts initial expectation: replacing despondence for purpose, silence for teaching, and isolation for teamwork—just as an intensive care unit repurposes urgency and gravity into meaning and hopefulness. It is this blending of emotional maturity, collaborative spirit, curiosity, and determination that creates an environment where the lessons of those who have come before empower and uplift all those present to learn from them, forging a legacy that serves both the living and the departed.

In all these varied environments, from the autopsy suite to the shared resident room, the common denominator is not morbidity, but meaning—the knowledge that our work, though often unseen, touches countless lives and leaves an indelible mark on us as practitioners.

Regardless of the rotation or service you are providing, whether in the autopsy suite or at your coffee-laden desk, there is a universal law: as time winds down towards the end of a long day, it is easy to slip into a state of complacency. Insidiously, it creeps in like an advancing fog, and much like the frog in the boiling water, you may not realize that you are losing focus until it has manifested significantly. It is in these moments that caution must be exercised; every slide and patient deserves your focus and attention, and when that wanes (as is human nature), it is critical to reset, take a break, and triage cases so that those that need increased scrutiny can be postponed to the next day. A helpful thing I like to ask myself is 'if this slide was from my family member or close friend, would I want someone like me in my current state to be determining their diagnosis?' By asking this question, we can avoid cursory examinations of cases that necessitate depth of reasoning and criticality. The human behind the cells, therefore, alludes to not only the patient but also the pathologist.

Although pathology is often associated with clinical detachment in those who are not enlightened as to its true nature, I hope these stories show the humanity that is present at its core. Behind every diagnosis is a person forever changed, and a pathologist who carries their stories with them.

Suggested Readings

1. Cocuz IG, Niculescu R, Popelea MC, Sabău A-H, Cocuz M-E, Manole M, et al. The emotional anatomy of diagnosis: a medical humanities approach to empathy in pathology. Diagnostics. 2025;15(15):1842 https://doi.org/10.3390/diagnostics15151842.
2. Ofri D. What doctors feel: how emotions affect the practice of medicine. Boston: Beacon Press; 2013.

9 The Path of the Imposter

When you enter medical school, buoyed by the aptitudes and capabilities you demonstrated during your undergraduate studies and interviews, it's easy to assume that the acquisition of knowledge will proceed at the same pace and structure as before. For me, undergraduate studies were straightforward: structured syllabi, prescribed course materials, and exams that tested a finite set of concepts. Success was measured by reading, understanding, and regurgitating material within clear boundaries. It was an assembly-line approach to learning—linear, predictable, and with definitive endpoints. But this system did little to prepare me for the vastness of medicine.

Medicine is not a finite body of knowledge; it is an ocean without shores. You can swim through its depths for years without ever glimpsing land. Trying to impose a rigid didactic structure on such an expansive field is not only impractical but counterproductive. Medicine's complexity defies simple cause-and-effect analysis. Concepts intertwine like threads in an intricate tapestry, creating a web of connections that cannot be compartmentalized. At the University of Alberta, our organ-based curriculum seemed linear at first glance—lectures on physiology, diseases, treatment strategies, and prognosis all tied neatly to a single organ system. I naively assumed that mastering one system would mean I had 'learned it all.' Once I had conquered the gastrointestinal system, I thought I knew everything about it. What I quickly realized was that medical

N. Pardell, *Scalpel, Scope, and Stain*,
https://doi.org/10.1007/978-3-032-25384-2_9

knowledge isn't linear; it's circular—or perhaps more accurately, it's like traversing an ever-expanding interconnected graph. Each node represents a concept or disease, and each edge signifies the connections between them.

This interconnectedness reflects the body itself. The exquisitely refined physiological systems of organs, tissues, and cells resist reductionist thinking. Diseases do not exist in isolation; they interact with their environments in ways that demand a holistic understanding. As I progressed in my training, I found myself revisiting concepts I thought I had mastered years earlier—only to discover new layers of complexity. It became clear that medical school provides the building blocks for understanding medicine, but residency is where those blocks are cemented together into a sturdy foundation. This 'glue' comes from experience: seeing the same concept repeatedly in different contexts until it becomes second nature.

Yet as we assemble our medical armamentarium, another phenomenon emerges—a voice from within that grows louder with each achievement. At first dismissible, this voice now begins to question your own competence: *Do you really belong here?* The more you learn, the more aware you become of what you don't know—and paradoxically, this growing awareness can make you feel less competent than before. This psychological paradox is what we call **Imposter Syndrome**, a pervasive yet under-discussed phenomenon in medicine.

Imposter Syndrome distorts your perception of competence and worthiness at every stage of training. From personal experience, I can tell you it's easy to feel like an imposter—even after years of study and accomplishment. To this day, I struggle with this cognitive bias. Swimming through an ocean of knowledge without signposts or lighthouses can leave you feeling as though you're treading water aimlessly leading to anxiety about whether you're truly prepared for the responsibilities ahead.

But these feelings are distortions—a trick of the mind borne from the vastness of knowledge itself. Imposter Syndrome can be reframed as evidence of growth rather than failure. Feeling like an imposter doesn't mean you're inadequate; it means you're striving for excellence in a field where perfection is unattainable but worth pursuing nonetheless. Growth is uncomfortable by nature—it forces us to confront our limitations—but it is also at the very heart of medicine.

By accepting lifelong learning as part of this journey, we can begin to see challenges not as signs of inadequacy but as milestones marking our progress. The very fact that we recognize these challenges means we've reached a point where we are capable of perceiving them—a testament to how far we've come rather than how far we have yet to go.

In pathology, I believe these feelings will come to a head before transitioning to independent practice. As of now, although I review cases and complete them as if they are my own, I still have significant oversight from the staff pathologists who are ultimately responsible for the case. I have never hit the button to publish the pathology report on the electronic medical record without review with my staff (and rightly so). This is similar to many stages of medical school clerkship and residency—there *should* be and *usually* is many layers above on which we operate. As a junior resident in my first year of off-service rotations, I logically understood that there were many safety nets above me that would catch my mishaps. However, emotionally, I felt that the life of the patient before me was inextricably dependent on my actions alone.

For example, I had a patient with very high blood pressure (hypertension) on my Internal Medicine rotation, one of my first rotations in first year residency. I started to sweat—there are numerous causes of hypertension that I thought I had to rule out. I was nervous, trying to recall every single cause of high blood pressure and what physical exam manoeuver I could do to ascertain them. I spent forever on this patient, thinking about renal (kidney) causes of hypertension like renal artery stenosis, masses like a pheochromocytoma, drug use such as cocaine, Cushing Syndrome, hyperthyroidism, among many others. Although I was generating a differential diagnosis, I was not focussing it on this specific patient or looking at probabilities. 'When you hear hoofbeats, think horses, not zebras,' is an old adage in medicine, and it has merit. Given the patient's context (medications, pre-existing medical conditions, age, etc.), and the likely culprits among all patients presenting with hypertension, all I had to ask was "did you take your blood pressure pill today?" to which the answer I most often received was "no, I forgot."

A simple solution to a common problem—adherence to prescribed medications. However, without the experience of having such failures, I would never come to realize what is likely and would never achieve any confidence in managing patients with nonspecific presentations such as 'high blood pressure,' or 'shortness of breath.' Similarly, in pathology, without readily accepting that I will make mistakes, I will never learn to become a good discerning pathologist. The challenge for us is maintaining our confidence and being proud of ourselves for the growth we showed. It is easy to forget these accomplishments and only focus on the next thing you have to do, but while the mentality of always striving for better is noble and desirable in this profession, one must be wary that it does not overshadow the self-confidence we have inevitably displayed in the past. This is one way in which we can tackle the voice inside our heads.

Starting out on general surgical pathology rotations, every case I received could be from a different organ—a thyroidectomy, a colon biopsy, a mucosal biopsy of the vocal cords, a hysterectomy with fallopian tubes and ovaries, etc. Each organ, with its constituent cell types and often unique pathologies, was overwhelming. For each tissue type, I felt the need to fully review all the normal histology of that organ, all of the possible diseases that could happen in this organ, and try to match what I'm seeing on the microscope to the images in the myriad books and online resources I had. This was unsustainable, as I had to sign the cases out in a reasonable timeframe! This feeling to understand everything *a priori* before looking at the case harkens back to my ability to retain all the PowerPoint slides in my mind's eye during undergraduate studies. It was a similar urge with the various resources at my disposal. I wanted to *read* everything before getting to *doing*. However, as I stated before, this is not feasible in medicine, and over time, I became more comfortable with the process of 'spot treatment,' looking up what I think I needed to know for that particular case at that particular time, forcing myself to leave the anxiety of leaving 7/8ths of the chapter unread that day behind. I tried to foster a mindset where I might gain one or two insights of knowledge into that organ system after reviewing with the staff pathologist, but not expecting to know everything the first time around, or the thirtieth. Sometimes you just have to start, and you can figure things out along the way, to avoid being paralyzed by the quantity of information. After seeing similar cases, more packets of knowledge build upon the prior, eventually coalescing into an amalgam better known as proficiency.

Suggested Readings

1. Franchi T, Russell-Sewell N. Medical students and the impostor phenomenon: a coexistence precipitated and perpetuated by the educational environment? Med Sci Educ. 2023;33(1):27–38.
2. McGaghie WC, Kristopaitis T. Deliberate practice and mastery learning: origins of expert medical performance. In: Cleland J, Durning SJ, editors. Researching medical education. Chichester (UK): Wiley Blackwell; 2015. Chapter 19.

Coffee, Cases, and Consults

10

When I was going through medical school, reflecting on my choice of specialty for the upcoming CaRMS matching process, I yearned to understand the day-in-the-life of the subsequent practitioners of the fields I was considering. I devoured YouTube videos, narrative medical books, and blog posts to vicariously situate myself within the respective domains. As I did this, I would assess my feelings as to the nature of the practice, the environment and collegiality therein, and the satisfaction I might take away from each day. As I stated at the beginning of this book, I only considered surgical specialties, but even among these there existed much variety. As I was applying for Anatomical Pathology in the second round of CaRMS, I employed the same investigative algorithm, trying to extract key information regarding the lifestyle, workload, clinical impact, and personal satisfaction that could be found in pathology.

The trouble is that many medical memoirs or medical narrative books focus on clinically oriented specialties. Internal medicine and surgical specialties dominate this literary landscape. I had trouble fully appreciating the intricacies of pathology, which lent itself to the trepidation I felt when I finally matched to the specialty. One of the goals of this book is to provide such a resource for medical students who might find themselves in the same shoes I once wore when determining their professional course. Pathology has a vast scope, but in this chapter, I will outline a typical day

N. Pardell, *Scalpel, Scope, and Stain*,
https://doi.org/10.1007/978-3-032-25384-2_10

on a general surgical pathology rotation, signing out cases whilst being part of the autopsy assignment and frozen section call. In addition, I will then outline a typical week on such a service, as different days would see the refinement of different skills, such as gross examination, and offer opportunities to participate in various forums such as the Academic Half-Day and multidisciplinary tumour boards. In doing this, I aim to extoll the collaborative culture and the balance afforded by the specialty upon you, the reader. I also want to stress the fact that no medical residency is easy; each has its stressors and demands good time management skills, albeit in different ways.

The day begins when I wake up at 6:45 A.M. I get ready for the day, quickly enjoy a morning coffee, and head out to the hospital, ensuring that my pager is clipped to my belt. A pager is that antediluvian relic hospital workers still carry—a chirping artifact from an era long past, pre-dating not only smartphones but possibly the invention of fire. It's like strapping a tiny, anxiety-inducing fossil to your belt, so you can be summoned in the most audacious and anachronistic way possible. Pagers are loud, and interrupt the burgeoning state of zen that accompanies the daily review of glass slides at precisely the right moment to halt the oncoming state of flow and replace it with dread. Exaggeration notwithstanding, pagers are old but allow anybody to contact you, whether you find yourself in the open air or the morgue surrounded by a concrete enclosure. Pagers are still used in pathology, to alert the wielder to incoming frozen sections (or intraoperative consultation as it is also known), or other clinicians with queries related to the laboratory.

By the time I've arrived and have myself seated at my assigned desk for the rotation, the clock strikes 8:00 A.M. I sip my second coffee of the day as I pull up the Operating Room (OR) slate on the computer, which denotes the scheduled patients that will be undergoing surgery that day. By reviewing 'the list,' I try to anticipate which operations might necessitate a frozen section so that I may look up the patient's clinical history, to provide context for the case should I get paged. I then inform the staff pathologist on frozen section call with me that I am present and will be joining them for any calls we receive. I check my email for any autopsies that are expected to come in for today and do the same investigative process. Autopsies at the university hospital are usually carried out in the mornings if all of the paperwork is received correctly and the personnel are available.

Next, I review my 'current cases' list on the Electronic Medical Record, to triage what cases I need to finish up, examine first, or those that I am still waiting for. Some of these cases may have carried over from prior days or are in the processing phase of the specimen's odyssey through the laboratory. Regardless of the case status, I make notes of each patient's clinical history, lab findings if relevant, and imaging reports so that I have context for the interpretation of the tissue slides when I transition to the microscope.

Assuming no autopsy planned for the morning, I then plan to spend a good portion of the morning and afternoon making diagnoses based on the tissue slides and writing the reports. During my slide review, I mark areas of interest, concern, and those with prognostic value for the patient on the slide with a coloured marker. Doing so facilitates learning when it comes to slide sign-out, or the review of the case with the staff pathologist I am assigned to. It not only shows that I recognized an abnormality, but provides a colourful reminder of what I might want clarified or seen with their more experienced eyes. As I am working through these cases, I may be showing select slides to other residents in the room for their opinion on the diagnosis, their opinion of what wording to use when drafting the report, or even for their education. We all show each other interesting cases to help one another out. Usually, these are high-yield cases for our licensing exam at the end of fourth year or something rare that not everyone comes across during residency. In doing so, we socialize, talk through pertinent points of whatever entity is currently being offered up for our spontaneous forums, and most importantly learn.

Between coffee runs and switching my Spotify playlist from 'Chopin' to 'Lo-Fi Study Beats,' I am reading textbooks and referencing the case findings with the vast repository of information online to help me arrive at an accurate diagnosis. In doing so I am learning more about the disease process I am seeing. This 'reading around your cases' approach is paramount to retaining the abundant characteristics of the near-innumerable entities encountered in medicine and pathology. Our brains thrive on visual information, and if the brain can associate the key facts of the disease with the visual information of the case readily seen through the microscope's optics, then you are more likely to retain that information. Next time I see the same entity, I might have to read the same key facts around it, but this repetition further consolidates the association between picture and knowledge. Such Hebbian plasticity is the basis of learning by association, and it is pervasively utilized in diagnostic specialties such as radiology and pathology where visual information and the need for pattern recognition are ubiquitous.

During the above process, I might receive zero to multiple pages from the laboratory. A number appears on my pager screen that I call back, to which they usually reply 'Frozen incoming.' I stop what I am doing, grab a protective gown and head downstairs to the OR, as the frozen section room is adjacent to this surgical habitat. Together with the staff covering the frozen section call, we process and stain the specimen (with great assistance from available technicians depending on the hospital site), and review the slides under the multiheaded microscope. The staff asks me about the clinical history of the patient (for example, if they have a biopsy-proven malignancy already), my opinion of the frozen section tissue slide, what I will tell the surgeon, and if satisfied, lets me call the operating theatre on the overhead speaker with the results.

Sometimes frozen sections can take 15 min, sometimes a couple of hours, depending on the number of specimens submitted by the surgeon and, if requested for margin assessment, due to the margin being repeatedly positive for cancer cells (thus necessitating further resection, and submission of further margins). Whilst in the intraoperative consultation room and cleaning the grossing station, I start to mentally review my 'to-do' list of the day; I may have some pending sign-out sessions with staff from the cases I was working on prior to getting called about this frozen section, more work-up to do regarding the cases on my desk, or having to juggle meeting times around multiple staff pathologists. Communication is of vital importance in medicine, and being proactive by letting your preceptors know the status of your shared work and plans for wrapping it up allows them to plan their schedule accordingly. In addition, everything runs smoother as expectations are managed, and by reaching out consistently, you show dependability and conscientiousness—desirable traits in a trainee.

Once back at my desk in the resident room, I resume whatever work was interrupted by the pager. This process might repeat multiple times in a day, and so task switching is an important skill in pathology. Once my cases are complete or I have ordered the appropriate ancillary tests, I review them with my assigned staff pathologist. We sit together at a double-headed microscope so we can both see the enigmatic biological world frozen in time on the glass slides. We go slide by slide, with their experiential eye correcting and educating my interpretations. Any marks I made on the slide are assessed, and a discussion usually ensues about the question I wanted to ask. After review, I go back to my desk, correct the report if warranted, and let them know it is finalized. If further testing was ordered and not received at the time, then that case usually waits until the next day to be signed out.

Before leaving for home around 5:00 p.m., a practice I have been trying to adopt is to make a list of the entities I saw that day that I was unfamiliar with, or that I need to review. This way I can directly consult my reference materials, 'read around the case,' and be more prepared for when I see it again. Having just seen the disease through the microscope, the retention of the minutiae and details of the entity will consolidate more readily into memory as I can now associate these facts with pictorial representations in my mind's eye.

Throughout the week, a similar workday algorithm applies. However, some days I must perform the gross examinations of specimens. By doing so, I learn what features are important to document and examine for a particular specimen or tissue type. Grossing is also the main way to generate the cases I will be seeing under the microscope. If I gross it, I examine it microscopically as well. Seeing a specimen throughout its voyage through the pathology department provides continuity, rounding out my understanding of the various roles within the laboratory.

Sprinkled throughout most weeks are various opportunities for didactic and case-based learning. With the surge of Zoom post-pandemic, most conferences and lectures are still done remotely, allowing anyone to log in from their respective and myriad locations. One of these didactic sessions runs for a whole morning, the Academic Half-Day. For the Anatomical Pathology residency, this is on

Tuesday mornings. Multiple hour-long sessions ensue covering various topics in pathology that run for a rolling 2-year curriculum. Some of these sessions are led by the residents, fostering teaching and presentation skills. Sometimes the lectures are not didactic but rather collaborative, an open forum to discuss residency concerns and wellness initiatives. Occasionally, sessions might also be conducted regarding life after residency as a staff physician, or touch on financial considerations for residents and staff.

In addition to the Half-Day sessions, there exist many opportunities to join various multidisciplinary tumour boards, where oncologists, radiologists, surgeons, radiation oncologists, and pathologists (among others) discuss challenging patient cases. After brief presentations by the constituent specialties regarding the patient case, a holistic and integrated approach to their management is sought. Does this patient need surgery, and if so, can the surgeon achieve a total resection? How many grays of radiation should this patient be afforded, taking into account their age, physical and mental fitness, and potential medical comorbidities? What should the clinician tell the patient as to their prognosis? These questions, and more, come up frequently. As a resident, you have an opportunity to participate in this collaborative effort. I have prepared some presentations for various patient cases pertaining to their pathology, replete with images of their tumour and attempted to distill the findings into a clear, cohesive explanation for the diagnosis my staff and I rendered. Seeing such an interdisciplinary approach rounds out your medical education, allowing you to experience the multiple considerations that are contemplated by a treatment team, especially in those fields outside your expertise.

Although many rotations, especially in the beginning of residency, focus on general surgical pathology of various organs and the ailments that commonly disease them, various *subspecialty* rotations exist in the later years. Rotations through dermatopathology, neuropathology, lymphoma pathology, breast pathology, genitourinary pathology, molecular pathology, cytology, and more help you focus your learning in the respective subdomain. Where breadth was the name of the game in the early years, depth is the focus in the later years. Throughout such rotations you can focus your studies, however you usually find that each subspecialty encompasses just as much vastness and complexity as any other. Much like a tree that iteratively branches into smaller and smaller segments, or arteries that branch into arterioles and then into capillaries, the field of medicine branches into various specialties (medical, surgical, diagnostic), and then into subspecialties. However, although the tree ends at the leaves, and the vasculature ends at the capillaries, each segment of the medical 'cascade' results in more subdivisions of equal scope, in a kind of epistemological fractal. You can never stop learning more in the health sciences, no matter how high your magnification is. Equally terrifying as it is awe-inspiring, a career in medicine is a pledge to continually evolve, adapt, learn, and integrate the ever-changing landscape of information. It is an oath to accept imperfection, but to strive towards its antithesis.

Suggested Readings

1. Price DW, Wang T, O'Neill TR, Morgan ZJ, Chodavarapu P, Bazemore A, et al. The effect of spaced repetition on learning and knowledge transfer in a large cohort of practicing physicians. Acad Med. 2025;100(1):94–102. https://doi.org/10.1097/ACM.0000000000005856.
2. Plotkin A, Olkhov-Mitsel E, Gagliardi AR. The impact of the pathologist in multidisciplinary cancer conferences on patient care: evidence from the literature. Am J Clin Pathol. 2023;159(4):352–7.

The Diagnostic Alliance

11

Modern medicine is increasingly characterized by specialization and further subspecialization, and at first glance, it would seem each field operates independently from one another. However, in reality, each discipline's spheres overlap and intersect in various ways, providing new perspectives and a synergy that allows a holistic picture of a patient's presentation than could be achieved within one domain itself. One of the most impactful overlaps Anatomical Pathology has with another medical discipline is that of Diagnostic Radiology. Both specialties operate largely outside the clinical curtain, outside the purview of direct patient contact, yet are inextricably linked to the patient's diagnostic odyssey through the hospital. These two specialties are complementary, acting as the foundation for accurate diagnosis and treatment decisions going forward. The parallels are unmistakable—the specialty that sees patterns in the light, and that which decodes them in shadow. Where radiology often provides a bird's-eye survey—the 'map' of disease—pathology supplies the up-close 'compass,' confirming, clarifying, or occasionally overturning the best guesses deduced from imaging. This dynamic, collaborative dialogue is particularly indispensable in bone and soft-tissue pathology, but its lessons reverberate throughout all medical disciplines and pathology subspecialties in particular.

Pathologists and radiologists are, at their core, diagnosticians, albeit from unique vantage points. Radiologists interpret anatomical

N. Pardell, *Scalpel, Scope, and Stain*,
https://doi.org/10.1007/978-3-032-25384-2_11

and functional changes in patients through various imaging modalities (ultrasound, computed tomography (CT), magnetic resonance imaging (MRI), positron emission tomography (PET), angiography, among others), providing essential descriptions of whatever pathological process is occurring in the patient's body, and generating various differentials to account for the patterns and relationships between structures seen. In this way, the radiologist acts as aerial reconnaissance, providing intelligence on the impact of the processes on the rest of the body. In contrast, the pathologist extracts information from the microscopic level of the disease processes, mostly at the local level/intrinsic to the disease itself.

It is easy to imagine that the boundaries of these specialties simply border one another, not crossing over into each others territory. However, it is the dialogue between them that provides crucial clarity and insight into the process as a whole and how it will affect the patient; insights that could not be gathered from one realm alone. Whether it's identifying the primary site of an enigmatic tumour, narrowing the differential for a perplexing mass, or correlating radiologic patterns with histopathologic architecture, their dialogue transforms ambiguity into clarity.

A radiologist may see particular patterns of grey and white and be confident enough to call a particular process outright. If and when a biopsy is warranted (usually for mass lesions), pathology then confirms what the radiologist surmised. Other times, the radiologist can only arrive at a differential diagnosis, as many entities can have similar appearances via imaging. When pathology receives a biopsy (often under image-guidance by radiologists!), they then refine the differential and often provide a definitive diagnosis.

A particular area of pathology that relies on radiologic correlation is bone and soft tissue pathology, a subspecialty that diagnoses various benign and malignant tumours of bone and the soft tissues (fat, muscle, nerve, fibrous tissue). Relatively rare tumours known as *sarcomas* are thereby diagnosed by these specialists. They work extremely closely with musculoskeletal radiologists, as the radiologic findings drastically impact the pathologic differential. For example, if a pathologist receives a bone biopsy without looking at the imaging (which one should never do), they might come up with a list of potential diagnoses based on the histologic appearance of the tissue. However, many entities appear similar in bone and soft tissue pathology, sometimes with only the subtlest of differences, and the pathologist relies heavily on the radiologic impression of the mass. Is it located in the middle of the femur (diaphysis), the transition between the end and the middle (metaphysis), or the end of the bone (epiphysis)? The radiologic appearance of the mass, the location in the bone, and the other characteristics noted in the imaging (periosteal reaction, cortical breakthrough, soft tissue extension, lytic versus sclerotic, etc.), not to mention patient demographics such as patient sex and age, greatly influence and refine the differential for the pathologist, such that an accurate diagnosis is reached. Particular cancers and benign lesions have characteristic appearances, or extremely probable locations from which they arise. For example, *osteosarcoma* classically involves the metaphysis, whereas *chondroblastoma* is seen in the epiphysis of young patients. A poignant example demonstrating the indispensable value of radiologic-pathologic correlation in bone tumour diagnosis is the case of *telangiectatic osteosarcoma* masquerading as an *aneurysmal bone cyst* (ABC). Under the microscope, both entities can appear quite similar: each displays prominent, blood-filled cystic spaces with septations, frequent multinucleated giant cells, and zones of reactive-looking bone. Without access to the clinical or radiological context, a pathologist examining a limited biopsy specimen may be misled by these overlapping features and erroneously diagnose a benign ABC, leading to a simple curettage by a surgeon without further treatment. However, the imaging characteristics might tell a different story. Imaging of telangiectatic osteosarcoma typically reveals ominous signs, such as aggressive, permeative bone destruction, cortical disruption, and the presence of a soft tissue mass adjacent to the bone lesion—findings that rarely, if ever, are seen in a true primary ABC, which more commonly shows a well-defined, expanding lesion that eats away at bone (known as lysis), with other features that disclose its benignity. Recognizing these discordant findings between scope and screen is crucial, as misclassifying these lesions can have dire consequences; an ABC is treated with curettage, whereas a telangiectatic osteosarcoma, being a highly malignant tumour, necessitates a wide resection by a surgeon and subsequent systemic chemotherapy. Thus, it is only by integrating clinical, radiologic, and histologic information that the pathologist can arrive at the correct, potentially life-saving diagnosis.

Radiologists, like pathologists, are not exempt from artifacts and alternative explanations for what they see on their screens. For example, in a patient with a bladder mass, radiologists can interpret different intensities of the surrounding tissues (bowel, uterus, etc.) to infer that a mass is invading into these structures, therefore meaning a more advanced stage of the process or lesion than that which maintains its local bounds. But just as in pathology, many visual interpretations of images can be explained by various other processes. For example, in a multidisciplinary tumour board, after the resection of a cancer, the radiologist often reviews the post-operative imaging after a specified time interval to then comment on an area of 'enhancement' within the surgical resection bed. The differential might includes a recurrence of the cancer, a portion of the mass left behind by the surgeon, or simply reactive and inflamed tissue, among other possible explanations. Clinical history and symptomatology, margin status decided by pathology, and other factors such as oncologic treatment and radiation oncologic treatment the patient received, can make one explanation more likely than others.

This diagnostic alliance plays out daily in multidisciplinary tumour boards, case conferences, and moments of collaborative problem-solving. The synergy between the specialty that images the whole and the other that examines the constituent parts leads to the most robust and nuanced understanding of each patient's condition. Their collaboration sets the stage for precision medicine, guiding multidisciplinary teams toward the best possible decisions for patients. In a multidisciplinary tumour board, where surgeons, radiation oncologists, medical oncologists, radiologists, and pathologists pool their expertise and direct it towards helping a particular patient, the feedback between radiology and pathology is essential. Radiologists identify and characterize lesions, estimate margins, and clarify patterns of spread or invasion for other members of the tumour board. Pathologists, in turn, analyze the tissue biopsies, explore differentials that arise from this analysis, assess and confirm margins microscopically, and suggest or confirm the identity of the process. The dialogue is iterative and synergistic; a radiologist may suspect malignancy based on aggressive imaging features, while the pathologist, with the glass slide in hand, may quell concern or take the differential down a markedly different path. Sometimes, the pathologist might request another biopsy to examine more tissue if imaging findings and histology do not correlate. Such feedback loops are essential in preventing overly narrow, context-blind diagnoses and maximizing diagnostic quality for each individual patient.

Frequently, in pathology, what is observed on imaging often mirrors what is revealed under the microscope. The radiologist's interpretation of structural patterns, or the levels of signal intensity in tissues, often finds its explanation in the cellular arrangements, microscopic changes, and results of ancillary stains seen by the pathologist. This corollary between radiologic and histologic findings not only aids diagnosis but also strengthens confidence in the decision-making of both disciplines and that of the patient-facing clinical team.

This relationship, where the imaging characteristics of lesions can be traced to distinct microscopic features, is evident in many disciplines of pathology. For example, in neuropathology, the radiographic appearance of a brain tumour can directly correlate with the histologic findings. In the case of *glioblastoma*, an extremely aggressive and lethal brain cancer, the radiologist might note a 'ring-enhancing lesion' (meaning that the gadolinium contrast agent given to the patient, used to aid resolution of tissues with MRI, is showing accumulation around the periphery of a mass) with central necrosis, and an infiltrative appearance of the lesion. Pathologically, the ring enhancement correlates with a microscopic finding known as *microvascular proliferation*—proliferative vessels/glomerular-like structures located at the edge of the tumour which are leaky, allowing fluid (plasma) and contrast to accumulate in the brain tissue. This explains the contrast 'enhancement' seen by the radiologist. The ill-defined outer 'boundary' of the tumour seen radiographically is also seen at the histological level—malignant cells infiltrate insidiously, covertly, and diffusely throughout the brain tissue, often obscured by intervening normal brain cells such that the precise boundary of the neoplasm is nearly impossible to derive.

Other pathology subspecialties also benefit from similar disciplinary crosstalk. For example, in thoracic pathology, the findings of 'ground-glass opacities' on CT scan of the lung elicit a broad differential. After the biopsy is received by pathology, they might see a lung adenocarcinoma in-situ, which has a particular pattern of spread through the lung tissue known as a 'lepidic' pattern. The cells that are malignant spread by using the lining of the lung airspaces (alveoli), rather than invading haphazardly through the lung tissue. It is known that a lepidic pattern can account for ground-glass opacity via CT, thus closing the loop and explaining the radiologic findings. In breast pathology, mammograms might identify calcifications in the breast, which also have a broad differential. On biopsy, a pathologist might see ductal carcinoma in-situ (a cancer that has not yet invaded, but is at high risk of doing so), which is often associated with calcifications. If the pathologist does not find calcifications to account for the radiology findings, further investigation must be done to find them, thereby seeking an explanation for the imaging findings. The pathologist might cut through the entire tissue block to search for the calcifications seen on imaging, sometimes even getting the tissue block X-rayed to confirm their presence. They might call the radiologist directly to discuss the discrepancy. Perhaps the biopsy missed capturing them, or perhaps two patient's biopsies were switched or mislabelled inadvertently in the laboratory. Correlation must be made between pathology and radiology for patient safety, accurate diagnosis, and quality assurance of each discipline. When extremely important decisions are to be made on radiologic and pathologic reports, precision and accuracy are tantamount, necessitating the diagnostic alliance.

The diagnostic alliance between radiology and pathology is more than simple correlation; it's a partnership grounded in shared curiosity, mutual respect, and common goals—the pursuit of providing clarity for patients. The radiologist provides the wide-reaching outline or topographical map of a disease process, charting the biological terrain in sweeping, grayscale vistas, while the pathologist ventures in close to examine the landmarks and landscape variations previously identified in high resolution. When these vantage points intersect—when map meets witness—we achieve the goal that modern medicine demands. That goal is precision.

As our fields evolve, and new technologies like artificial intelligence, advanced molecular analysis, and digital pathological workflows weave their way into daily practice, the territory between disciplines grows ever more blurred. Far from replacing the human intuition or the necessity of dialogue, these innovations will likely enrich our diagnostic acumen and decrease our margins of error. They promise increased correlation between shadow and substance—between the macroscopic patterns that radiologists see and the microscopic realities that pathologists uncover.

At the centre of all this collaboration, and all these advances, remains the patient. It's easy to lose sight of that fact amid all the data and digital images, but ultimately every consult, every tumour board debate, and every nervous phone call to clarify a finding is about providing patients—and their families—with the understanding, guidance, and hope they deserve.

So, as we move forward, it's worth remembering that the best medicine is practiced when we share perspectives, challenge each other's assumptions, and look together through the lens and across the screen. Because only then do we truly see the whole picture—one that no single viewpoint, no matter how skilled, could ever capture alone.

Suggested Readings

1. Kuo MD, Yamamoto S. Next generation radiologic-pathologic correlation in oncology: Rad-Path 2.0. AJR Am J Roentgenol. 2011;197(4):990–7. https://doi.org/10.2214/AJR.11.7163.
2. Sorace J, Aberle DR, Elimam D, Lawvere S, Tawfik O, Wallace WD. Integrating pathology and radiology disciplines: an emerging opportunity? BMC Med. 2012;10:100. https://doi.org/10.1186/1741-7015-10-100.

Conclusion

12

While surgeons wield scalpels to exhume disease from patients, pathologists equip lenses, stains, and ancillary laboratory tests to extract vital diagnostic information for patients. Operating at the crossroads between medicine and humanity, pathologists are not exempt from the patient experience. The lifeblood of pathology revolves around patient care, despite the stereotypical depictions of pathology as a specialty relegated outside the scope of human interaction. Whether signing out cases that will directly impact patient lives both medically and socially, and their continued management by other clinicians, pathologists are an instrumental element in almost every patient's course throughout the medical system, intimately annealed to the care provided by other physicians and allied health professionals.

Pathologists have many specialized tools to arrive at their conclusions, which are often seen as infallible even to other medical specialties. Although it is true that pathology offers some of the highest precision when it comes to diagnosis, the specialty is, as most are in medicine, both an art and a science. Objectivity reigns supreme, exemplified by the burgeoning research on the incorporation of artificial intelligence solutions, computational pathology and digital pathology workflows, but due to the human behind the microscope, an element of subjectivity remains. This subjectivity might seem like a downside on the surface, but it is paramount when

N. Pardell, *Scalpel, Scope, and Stain*,
https://doi.org/10.1007/978-3-032-25384-2_12

it comes to difficult cases with artifacts, an unusual clinical history, or a morphology that might not match the supervised training set for a machine learning algorithm. The ability to share cases and collaborate with other colleagues and physicians in the care of the patient is of utmost importance to arrive at diagnostic accuracy. It is this amalgamation of context and other opinions that one can reach the highest levels of diagnostic precision. The landscape of pathology will continue to transform with advances in molecular diagnostics, digital pathology, and artificial intelligence, and these innovations promise to enhance our diagnostic capabilities. Moreover, they will also demand adaptability and a commitment to lifelong learning. As residents, trainees, and future pathologists, we are uniquely positioned to embrace these changes, advocate for our specialty, and contribute to the advancement of patient care.

One of the most pivotal things I have learned through this journey (and continue to learn until I complete my residency) is that pathologists are not devoid of human interaction or human connection. Every case or autopsy is a patient and should be afforded not only a portion of your time but also that of your soul. It is easy to become inundated with work and focus on the task at hand, and often this is necessary. But if we do not look back and reflect on the especially poignant cases to understand how they made us feel, then we cannot minimize the loss of our own humanity.

As much as compassion is essential to medical specialties, so too is resilience. Assaults on identity in the form of imposter syndrome come from within, while batteries aimed at our emotions originate from the cases, diseases, and patient stories dealt with every day. Balancing emotional toll and occupational duty is a constant decree demanded of medical professionals, maintaining their humanity while encouraging optimal patient care.

The challenges faced in residency—moments of uncertainty, imposter syndrome, and the unrelenting breadth of knowledge to master—are not signs of inadequacy, but rather the very crucible in which adaptability, precision, and wisdom are forged. It is natural to feel overwhelmed at times, but within each challenge lies an invaluable opportunity for growth and discovery. The evolving landscape of pathology, with its integration of molecular techniques, digital platforms, and artificial intelligence, reminds us that learning is not a finite endeavour. Instead, it is a lifelong commitment—one that rewards curiosity, resilience, and a willingness to embrace change.

If you, the reader, are a medical student seeking information on pathology and its inner workings, then I hope you gained insight into the compelling and fascinating world I now call home. I hope that the discussion on differential diagnoses, the insights and emotional aspects of patient cases, and the understanding of the inter-relationship between diagnostic medicine and clinical medicine can be carried forward with you into whatever specialty you choose. If you picked up this book for pure interest, then I hope I have achieved that goal, shining a light on a profession that is not well known.

My journey in pathology is still unfolding. The lessons I've gathered during residency—sometimes hard-won, but always meaningful—are just the groundwork for a career of ongoing learning, discovery, and service. I owe a deep debt of gratitude to the mentors who have guided me, the colleagues who have challenged and supported me, and the patients whose stories have given purpose to every case. As I move forward, I'm reminded that the pathologist's lens isn't just a diagnostic tool—it's a way of seeing the intricate stories written in tissue, the patterns of health and disease that define our lives. Residency has shown me that curiosity, teamwork, and empathy are every bit as essential as technical skill. Pathology may not always be in the spotlight, but it is truly the bedrock of modern medicine. For those who share a fascination with the 'why' behind disease, who are energized by problem-solving and the thrill of discovery, I hope these pages have offered insight, reassurance, and a sense of community. The future of pathology is exciting, driven by innovation, collaboration, and the passion of those who look deeper. Here's to continuing the journey: to learning, teaching, and making a difference—one slide at a time.

Appendix A: Glossary

Term Description

Academic Half-Day Scheduled block of time, typically one morning per week, dedicated to didactic and case-based learning for residents, covering a rolling curriculum of specialty topics.

Adnexal Tumors Tumours arising from skin appendages such as hair follicles, sebaceous glands, or sweat glands.

Amelanotic Describes a lesion (often melanoma) lacking melanin pigment, making it appear non-pigmented.

Ancillary Studies Additional laboratory tests performed on tissue specimens, such as immunohistochemistry, molecular testing (e.g., PCR, NGS), or special stains, used to aid in diagnosis.

Anhidrosis Absence of sweating, often due to loss of sympathetic innervation.

Atypia Abnormal appearance of cells, often referring to nuclear size, shape, or staining, which may indicate malignancy.

Autopsy A post-mortem examination performed to determine the cause of death, study disease processes, and provide quality assurance and education.

Basal Cell Carcinoma A common type of skin cancer arising from the basal cells of the epidermis.

Benign Describes a tumour or growth that does not invade surrounding tissues or metastasize; generally considered non-cancerous.

Biopsy A medical procedure involving the removal of tissue for diagnostic examination under a microscope.

Carcinoma A malignant tumour arising from epithelial cells.

N. Pardell, *Scalpel, Scope, and Stain*,
https://doi.org/10.1007/978-3-032-25384-2

CaRMS (Canadian Residency Matching Service) A national matching system in Canada that pairs medical students with residency programs based on mutual rankings.

Chief Cells (Parathyroid) One of the main cell types in the parathyroid gland is responsible for producing parathyroid hormone.

Clear Cell Descriptive term for cells with clear cytoplasm, often seen in certain tumours like clear cell renal cell carcinoma.

Clinical-Pathological Correlation The process of integrating clinical information with pathological findings to arrive at a diagnosis.

Clone (in cancer context) A group of cells within a tumour sharing a common ancestor and set of genetic mutations.

Congenital A condition present at birth, due to genetic or developmental factors.

Consultation (in pathology) Review and discussion of a case with another pathologist or clinical team for diagnostic clarification or confirmation.

Cryotome A device used to cut thin sections of frozen tissue for microscopic examination during frozen section procedures.

Cytology The study of individual cells and their characteristics often used in cancer screening and diagnosis.

Dedifferentiation The process by which cells lose their specialized characteristics often associated with high-grade tumours.

Desmoplastic Melanoma A rare variant of melanoma characterized by spindle-shaped cells and a fibrous stroma, often lacking pigment and mimicking scars or other benign lesions.

Differential Diagnosis A systematic list of possible diseases or conditions that could explain a patient's symptoms or tissue findings, ranked by likelihood.

Discordant Describes findings that do not match between two investigative modalities (e.g., imaging and histology), indicating possible error or complexity in diagnosis.

Eosinophilic Secretions Pink-staining material within cells or glands, often seen in certain tumours under H&E stain.

Epigenetic Referring to modifications that alter gene expression without changing the DNA sequence, often implicated in cancer development.

Epidermis The outermost layer of the skin.

Frozen Section A rapid intraoperative pathology technique where tissue is quickly frozen, sectioned, stained, and examined to provide immediate diagnostic information to surgeons.

Fibroid (Leiomyoma) A benign smooth muscle tumour of the uterus, often causing abnormal bleeding or pain.

Fixation (tissue context) The process of preserving tissue using chemicals (e.g., formalin) to prevent decay and maintain structure for microscopy.

FISH (Fluorescence In Situ Hybridization) A molecular cytogenetic technique used to detect and localize the presence or absence of specific DNA sequences on chromosomes.

Forensic Pathology A subspecialty of pathology focused on determining the cause of death in medico-legal cases, including sudden, unexpected, or violent deaths.

Germ Cell Neoplasm A tumour derived from germ cells, most commonly arising in the gonads (testis, ovary), but also occurring in extragonadal locations.

Gross Examination (Grossing) The process of visually inspecting and describing surgical specimens, taking measurements, and selecting tissue for microscopic analysis.

Hallmarks of Cancer Fundamental traits shared by most cancers: sustained proliferative signalling, evasion of growth suppressors, resistance to cell death, replicative immortality, angiogenesis, invasion, metastasis, metabolic reprogramming, and immune evasion.

Hematoxylin and Eosin (H&E) Stain The standard stain used in pathology to visualize tissue architecture: hematoxylin stains nuclei blue, and eosin stains cytoplasm pink.

Histopathology The microscopic study of diseased tissue.

Immunohistochemistry (IHC) A laboratory technique using antibodies to detect specific antigens in tissue sections, aiding in the identification and classification of cells and tumours.

Intraoperative Consultation A real-time diagnostic service provided by pathologists during surgery, often using frozen section analysis, to guide surgical decision-making.

Iatrogenic A problem or condition caused by medical examination or treatment.

Leiomyosarcoma A malignant tumour of smooth muscle origin.

Lesion An area of abnormal tissue change due to disease or injury.

Line of Differentiation The cell lineage or type from which a tumour arose, as determined by morphology or ancillary studies.

Lymph Node A small, bean-shaped structure that is part of the lymphatic system and plays a role in immune response; often evaluated for metastasis in cancer.

Malignant Describes a tumour that invades surrounding tissues and has the potential to metastasize (spread to distant sites); cancerous.

Margin (Surgical Margin) The edge or border of tissue removed during surgery; assessed to determine if disease (e.g., cancer) has been completely excised.

Melanoma A malignant tumour of melanocytes, the pigment-producing cells of the skin.

Metastasis The spread of cancer cells from the original (primary) site to distant organs or tissues.

Mitotic Figures Cells in the process of division (mitosis), visible under the microscope; increased numbers often indicate rapid cell proliferation, as seen in malignancy.

Molecular Diagnostics Laboratory techniques used to analyze DNA, RNA, or proteins to detect mutations or alterations driving disease, especially in cancer.

Morphology The form and structure of cells and tissues, as observed under the microscope.

Neoplasm An abnormal growth of tissue, which can be benign or malignant (cancerous); literally means 'new growth.'

Necrosis Unregulated cell death resulting in tissue breakdown; often seen in rapidly growing tumours that outstrip their blood supply.

Neoplastic Pertaining to or characteristic of neoplasms (tumours).

Neutrophils A type of white blood cell involved in acute inflammation and defence against infection.

Nucleolus A small, dense body within the nucleus, often enlarged and prominent in cancer cells.

Oncocytic Describes cells with an abundant, granular, eosinophilic cytoplasm rich in mitochondria, often seen in tumours of various organs.

Oxyphil Cells (Parathyroid) A cell type in the parathyroid gland with abundant eosinophilic cytoplasm; its function is not fully understood.

Parathyroid Gland Small glands located near or within the thyroid, responsible for regulating calcium levels via parathyroid hormone.

Pathogenesis The mechanism by which a disease develops, from initial cause to final effects.

Pathologists' Assistant (PA) A trained professional who assists pathologists in the gross examination and processing of surgical specimens and autopsies.

Perineural Invasion Cancer cells seen tracking along or invading nerves are often a sign of aggressive disease.

Pleomorphic Describes variability in the size and shape of cells or their nuclei, often seen in malignancy.

Prussian Blue (Perl's) Stain A special stain used to detect iron in tissues, often to confirm the presence of asbestos bodies or hemosiderin.

Prognosis The likely outcome or course of a disease; the chance of recovery or recurrence.

Proliferation Cell growth and division; increased proliferation is a hallmark of cancer.

Prostatic Adenocarcinoma A malignant tumour arising from the glandular tissue of the prostate.

Radiologic-Pathologic Correlation The process of aligning and comparing imaging findings with pathology results to refine or confirm the diagnosis.

Replicative Immortality The ability of cancer cells to divide indefinitely, often by activating telomerase or alternative lengthening mechanisms.

Sarcoma A malignant tumour arising from connective tissues such as bone, muscle, or fat.

Signet Ring Cell A type of cell with a large vacuole that displaces the nucleus to one side, seen in certain aggressive cancers such as gastric or colon signet ring cell carcinoma.

Spindled Cells Cells that are elongated and tapered at both ends are often seen in sarcomas and certain variants of melanoma.

Squamous Cell Carcinoma A common type of skin cancer arising from squamous epithelial cells, can also occur in other organs.

Storiform Pattern A pattern of fibrosis or tumour growth resembling a cartwheel or mat, often seen in certain tumours or fibrosing conditions.

Subclone A genetically distinct population of cells within a tumour, arising from further mutations and selection.

Telomerase An enzyme that maintains telomere length and is often reactivated in cancer cells, conferring immortality.

Tumor Board A multidisciplinary meeting where complex cancer cases are discussed by a team of specialists to determine optimal management.

Tumor Microenvironment The surrounding cells, stroma, blood vessels, and immune environment in which a tumour exists, affecting its growth and response to therapy.

Vascular Relating to blood vessels; often used in the context of causes of disease (e.g., vascular causes of jaundice).

VITAMIN CDE Mnemonic Memory aid for constructing a differential diagnosis by etiology: Vascular, Infectious/inflammatory, Trauma/toxin, Autoimmune/allergic, Metabolic, Iatrogenic/idiopathic, Neoplastic, Congenital, Degenerative, Endocrine.

Warburg Effect A metabolic shift in cancer cells toward aerobic glycolysis (producing energy from glucose even in the presence of oxygen); favours biomass production over ATP efficiency.

Appendix B: Anatomical Pathology Subspecialties

Dermatopathology

The focus of Dermatopathology is on all disease processes related to the skin, nail, mucous membranes, hair, and subcutaneous tissue. Diseases can be either primarily affecting these structures or secondary to systemic pathologies. They deal with neoplastic entities like melanoma, squamous cell carcinoma, and various tumours of hair follicles, sweat glands and other dermal appendages, as well as autoimmune and inflammatory conditions like vasculitis, lupus, and psoriasis. Dermatopathologists rely heavily on clinicopathologic correlation—a good understanding of medical dermatology and the differentials considered by dermatologists help inform the pathologic differential, as many entities can overlap histologically. Pro-tip: Always check the clinical history and tailor your differential to the clinical suspicions. Keep a broad outlook, and remember that many disease processes can affect the skin even if it isn't localized to the skin itself.

N. Pardell, *Scalpel, Scope, and Stain*,
https://doi.org/10.1007/978-3-032-25384-2

Neuropathology	A separate residency in Canada. Encompasses the diagnosis of pathologies occurring in the central nervous system (brain, spinal cord), peripheral nerves, neuromuscular junction and muscles themselves, with a focus on tumours, neurodegenerative diseases, demyelinating conditions, and potentially forensic neuropathology. Neuropathologists handle brain biopsies and tumour resections, utilize intraoperative smears at the time of frozen section, and examine the nervous system during autopsies. The specialty is intimately aligned with molecular pathology for diagnostic and even prognostic purposes. Common cases include the diagnosis of various gliomas, meningiomas, metastatic tumours to the brain and spinal cord, and infections. Pro-tip: Know the latest WHO CNS classifications, keep up to date with c-IMPACT publications, and always correlate biopsy findings with neuroimaging.
Breast Pathology	Branch of pathology that deals with benign and malignant breast diseases such as fibroadenomas, ductal and lobular breast carcinoma, Paget's Disease of the nipple, and mastitis. They evaluate core needle biopsies, resections, and sentinel lymph nodes, as well as hormonal markers (HER2, ER, PR) for prognostic and predictive information (such as eligibility for certain drugs). Pro-tip: Always correlate with imaging studies, carefully quantitate margin status and the extent of in-situ carcinoma, and document findings thoroughly for optimal patient care.

Gynecologic Pathology	Deals with diseases of the female genital tract, including the uterus, fallopian tubes, ovaries, and supporting structures (broad ligament, etc.), seeing biopsies and large resections. Frozen section consultation is frequent, especially for ovarian tumours and during staging procedures. Typical pathologies include cervical dysplasia, endometrial carcinoma, leiomyoma (fibroids), gestational trophoblastic disease, and ovarian tumours. Pro-tip: Know your classification and grading systems, be diligent in documenting the extent that a tumour involves the ovarian surface and tubes, and check if the specimen was received into the lab intact or ruptured intraoperatively, as this can have staging consequences.
Genitourinary Pathology	Covers prostate, bladder, ureters, kidneys, and male reproductive organs. They evaluate biopsies, transurethral resections, large resections (nephrectomies, cystoprostatectomies, etc.) and cytological preparations. Common entities encountered include prostatic and urothelial carcinomas, renal cell carcinomas, and testicular tumours. Medical renal pathology is also a distinct subspecialty dealing with non-neoplastic diseases of the kidney (pyelonephritis, autoimmune diseases, and glomerulonephritides, amyloidosis, renal transplant assessment, etc.) Pro-tip: Be diligent in calculating the extent of involvement of prostate cancer on biopsies, master Gleason grading, and keep abreast of newly developing tumour entities considering the surge of molecular integration into diagnosis.

Pulmonary Pathology	Pulmonary pathology focuses on the lungs and mediastinal structures. They handle biopsies and resections (wedge resections, lobectomies) for lung nodules and masses, as well as often interpret cytologic preparations such as bronchoalveolar lavage, bronchial washings/brushings, and endobronchial ultrasound-guided biopsies of mediastinal lymph nodes. Sometimes, they may see lung explants due to interstitial lung diseases, and assess the status of transplanted lungs. Common pathologies include infection/inflammatory entities such as tuberculosis, sarcoidosis, and granulomatosis with polyangiitis (a vasculitis), as well as oncologic entities such as adenocarcinoma, small cell carcinoma, and metastatic tumours. Medical lung pathology includes the spectrum of interstitial lung disease such as hypersensitivity pneumonitis and usual interstitial pneumonia (the histologic pattern often correlating to clinically diagnosed idiopathic pulmonary fibrosis). Pro Tip: Know the molecular changes of lung adenocarcinoma and what molecular testing is available for advanced-stage cases. Also, ensure you rule out metastatic disease before assigning a primary lung cancer diagnosis, especially if the clinical history is ambiguous or they have a prior history of distant cancer.
Head & Neck Pathology	Involves the oral cavity, larynx, salivary glands, thyroid, and parathyroid, typically dealing with biopsies, resections, and intraoperative consultations. Common entities include squamous cell carcinoma and its subtypes, papillary thyroid carcinoma, pleomorphic adenoma, and parathyroid adenoma. Pro-tip: Master cytopathology classification systems, correlate with imaging (head and neck anatomy is one of the most complex regions of the body), and learn the sometimes subtle differences between thyroid entities.

Gastrointestinal Pathology and Hepatobiliary pathology	Vast specialty dealing with the entire GI tract, liver, and pancreas, bile ducts and gallbladder, working with biopsies and resections (sometimes multi-organ such as Whipple specimens), cytology, and sometimes transplants. Oncologic and medical diseases are both prominent in these organs. Esophagitis, colon and stomach adenocarcinomas, inflammatory bowel disease, GI lymphomas, hepatitis, hemochromatosis, A1AT deficiency, hepatocellular carcinoma, cholangiocarcinoma, and pancreatic ductal carcinoma are only a few of the entities commonly encountered. Pro-tip: Always utilize mapping diagrams for gross examination, review endoscopy, and keep a broad differential when working up cases. Master grading for cirrhosis, chronic hepatitis, and overlap syndromes in the liver.
Hematopathology	A separate residency in Canada. Specializes in diseases of bone marrow, lymph node, spleen, and blood, especially lymphomas and leukemias (Lymphoma pathology can be practiced after a fellowship if coming from Anatomical Pathology). Practitioners may assess biopsies from lymph nodes and bone marrow, as well as analyze results from flow cytometry, cytogenetic studies, immunohistochemistry, and advanced molecular tests. Common entities (there are many) include Hodgkin lymphoma, follicular lymphoma, Burkitt Lymphoma, Diffuse large B-cell lymphomas, various leukemias, multiple myeloma, histiocytosis, and myelodysplastic syndrome. Hematopathologists are adept at integrating the complexity of various modalities, including light microscopic descriptions of morphology, ancillary studies, and frequently changing classification systems, making diagnosis quite challenging. Pro-tip: Keep up-to-date with WHO and ICC classifications and always synthesize results from multiple modalities (surgical pathology, flow cytometry, etc.) for accurate diagnosis.

Bone & Soft Tissue Pathology	Covers neoplastic and non-neoplastic diseases of mesenchymal tissue (e.g., bone, nerve, fat, muscle, fibrous tissue) working with biopsies, wide local resections, and even amputations. This subspecialty has a rich integration with molecular pathology, especially to detect characteristic gene fusions that often define entities. Radiologic correlation is frequent to narrow differentials and ensure accuracy. As well, this specialty deals with entities that are relatively rare compared to most other pathology subspecialties (sarcomas make up around 1% of all cancer diagnoses). Some encountered entities include osteosarcoma, Ewing sarcoma, liposarcoma, gastrointestinal stromal tumour, solitary fibrous tumour, desmoid fibromatosis, malignant peripheral nerve sheath tumours, and osteoid osteoma. The rarity, morphologic overlap, and often small biopsy specimens introduce diagnostic risks and pitfalls. Pro-tip: Always correlate with imaging and use extended ancillary panels (IHC and molecular) for unusual or poorly differentiated tumours. Cement your knowledge of the biologic potential for local invasion and/or metastasis in various tumours, and master the use of tailored IHC panels.
Pediatric/Perinatal/ Placental Pathology	Covers diseases of infancy, childhood, fetus, and placenta, with a workflow including pediatric biopsies, fetal/infant autopsies, placenta examination, and genetic/molecular testing. Wilms' tumour, neuroblastoma, medulloblastoma, congenital anomalies, celiac disease, Hirschsprung's disease, and placental infarct or infection are typical. Challenges stem from rare 'zebra' entities, processes that are unique to younger age groups or present at an early age, and high emotional toll (especially in autopsy examinations). The subspecialty works with pediatricians, neonatologists, maternal-fetal, and genetic teams. Pro-tip: Use age-based reference ranges, respect unique gross anatomy, and communicate sensitively in difficult cases.

Cytopathology Diagnoses based on individual/small cell samples, such as Pap smears, FNAs, and fluid cytology. Applies stains, IHC, molecular/FISH, and rapid on-site evaluation for adequacy (ROSE). Pap abnormalities, thyroid nodules, metastatic carcinoma, and infectious/inflammatory processes are most common. Artifacts and sampling limitations introduce uncertainty, especially when reporting indeterminate categories. Interacts with radiologists, surgeons, and clinical services performing procedures. Pro-tip: Know specimen adequacy criteria, correlate with the corresponding tissue sample, and always recommend repeat sampling if in doubt or if results are equivocal.

Molecular Pathology Applies genomic/molecular methods such as PCR, NGS, and FISH to tissue and cytology samples for mutation testing, translocation assessments, and the determination of gene signatures. Some targets and tests include KRAS, EGFR, BRCA, MSI testing, and the identification of numerous fusion genes. Interpreting variants-of-unknown-significance, dealing with tissue exhaustion, and rapidly evolving technology are key challenges. The subspecialty collaborates with oncology, genetics, and all diagnostic/treatment subspecialties. Pro-tip: Conserve tissue for molecular testing, consider splitting tissue samples into multiple blocks, and stay current with your institution's testing menu and panel indications.

Forensic Pathology Applies autopsy pathology to legal and investigative settings (cause/manner of death, trauma, sudden infant death). The workflow includes external exam, full autopsy, toxicology, and radiology with legal documentation. Blunt and penetrating trauma, overdose, homicide, sudden natural deaths, and child abuse are common findings. Emotional distress, detailed documentation, and legal/court interactions add difficulty. Works closely with police, social services, and legal systems. Pro-tip: Be meticulous with documentation and evidence, and maintain a routine of self-care given the emotional toll.

Appendix C: Common Pitfalls and Pearls in Pathology Residency

Having been in pathology residency for 4 years (as of this writing), I have had to create, adapt, and ultimately extensively revise my approaches to all things, including communication with colleagues, drafting of concise, well-written and informative reports, as well as how to tackle the largely self-directed learning in the face of daunting amounts of information. This appendix outlines common pitfalls and biases one easily makes in the beginning years of pathology residency, and pearls from my own experiences that might resonate with future pathology residents. In so doing, I hope to ease the transition from predominantly clinical acumen to foster diagnostic considerations. Keep in mind that these are my experiences and perspectives, and a one size-fits-all approach might be unrealistic. Nevertheless, I hope the lessons I have learned will at least illuminate the scope of the daily challenges a pathologist-in-training might face.

N. Pardell, *Scalpel, Scope, and Stain*,
https://doi.org/10.1007/978-3-032-25384-2

Common Pitfalls in Pathology Residency

A. Diagnostic Pitfalls

Over-reliance on morphology alone: the danger of 'pattern-matching' without clinical/radiological context.	Many entities can mimic one another—always review the clinical and radiologic impressions as well as patient demographics (age, sex, family history, etc.) as these can hone your differential. Also, be aware of the many patterns and histologic findings of other entities that could account for what you see under the microscope (Example: basal cell carcinoma versus basaloid squamous cell carcinoma versus basosquamous carcinoma)
Underutilization (or overordering) of ancillary studies such as IHC and molecular tests.	IHC should not be used in a 'shotgun' approach, seeing what sticks. It should always be used to answer a diagnostic question. Because no marker or test is 100% sensitive or specific, be prepared to back up your IHC panel or molecular assay proposal with valid diagnostic reasons for their ordering. By ordering too few tests (depending on the case), you run the risk of missing entities masquerading as one another, or missing important predictive and prognostic information for clinicians (MMR testing in colon cancer, HER2 testing in breast cancer for Herceptin therapy considerations)
Missing the 'zebra' by assuming all cases are routine.	As your knowledge grows, you will come to appreciate the histologic overlap of many entities, including rare ones. You can only rule something out if you know it exists! Conversely, assuming all 'generic' cases are zebras will also lead to overuse of IHC markers used to chase them. Clinical and radiologic correlation is essential!
Not recognizing artifacts or mistaking them for pathology.	With time and knowledge of general pathologic principles, you will be able to make 'on-the-fly' decisions about if what you are seeing is a pathologic process, an artifact of laboratory processing, or a variation of normal histology. You must recognize 'normal' before being able to resolve the 'abnormal'!

B. Workflow and Time Management

Failing to triage cases by complexity and urgency.	By understanding which diseases need prompt diagnosis so that management teams can enact therapy is crucial. Don't let the lymphoma diagnosis sit on your desk while you sign out the regular colon polyps!
Procrastinating on grossing or report writing; letting 'small' tasks pile up.	Your work comes from that of the pathologists you are assigned to. They will appreciate the comprehensive review you've done of the case with expediency. The lab tracks turnaround-time, an important metric that staff pathologists keep in mind not only for their performance reviews but also to ensure patients and their clinicians get the important answers they need promptly.
Inadequate preparation for signout with staff.	Do not fall into the trap when dealing with a hard case to just let your staff handle it—One day, it will be you making the important decisions (and clicking the important button to publish the report), so by doing your best and being honest with what you have questions and concerns about, you maximize your learning and build proficiency for when you become an independent practitioner. Also, your effort reflects on you as a learner and future colleague. Residency is a 5-year (in Canada) job interview!

C. Professionalism and Communication

Not seeking help or a second opinion when unsure.	Always mark areas on slides you have questions about to review with your staff, and utilize your peers for their opinions and perspectives on your case if you have difficulty. Collaboration is a part of the profession, so don't feel intimidated by seeking help! At the end of the day, it's all to provide an accurate diagnosis for a patient who needs it.
Poor documentation—incomplete or rushed reports.	Residency can be busy, and everybody understands this. Be honest about your workload, and always give each case the attention it's due. If all else fails, ensure you've reviewed the slides, so that after review with your staff, you can quickly finalize the report for sign-out.
Overlooking the importance of intradepartmental consultations	It is commonplace to show cases that are difficult or have diagnostic ambiguity to colleagues for their opinions, to ensure the diagnosis is correct or even to be confident in communicating the uncertainty with the clinical team in a comment on your report. There is strength in numbers—try not to act as a lone wolf, as this can sometimes lead to harmful consequences for the patient.

D. Wellbeing and Attitude

Neglecting self-care and social connection due to solitary or busy periods.	Taking deliberate time to support your own mental health and wellness is essential in medicine. By proactively setting aside space in your schedule for activities that restore your energy and bring you satisfaction, you help safeguard against burnout and maintain the resilience needed to serve patients for years to come. Prioritizing rest and renewal isn't just self-care—it's a strategic investment in your ability to provide excellent, sustainable care over the long term.
Allowing imposter syndrome to sap confidence rather than fuel improvement.	Many residents grapple with perfectionism. Remember that there is a reason you are in a training program—you are not expected to be functioning at the level your brain is demanding of you at the current time. Instead of personal beratement, celebrate the wins and learn from the losses so you can do better next time; that is the true expectation. Perfection is the enemy of good.

Pearls and Strategies for Success

A. Diagnostic Approach

Always correlate: check clinical and imaging data before and during review.	Clinicoradiologic correlation is essential to provide context for the patient presentation, which is vital for building differential diagnoses. As well, your staff will expect you to be versed in the patient history and imaging findings before you sign out with them for the same reason. After all, diagnosticians are fully trained medical doctors and have to endure the gauntlet of medical school for many reasons, not the least of which is that it grounds their specialized expertise in basic medical principles to provide a holistic picture of a patient and their problems.

Build differentials **systematically** using mnemonics or algorithms.	Systems, algorithms, and checklists are ubiquitous in medicine and other professions where errors come at high costs (aviation, military operations, nuclear power industry, construction engineering, space agencies). By following strict systematic assessments, diagnosticians reduce human error while maximizing patient safety. As well, in performing systematic assessments, you ensure that you have considered all possibilities for a given case—critical to ensure accurate and defendable diagnosis and catching of the occasional 'zebra'!
Pause and reflect: if a case feels 'off,' step back and re-examine.	Trust your intuition, especially as your expertise and knowledge accumulate. Your brain is parsing information unconsciously, and when the clinical, radiologic and pathologic variables don't seem to complement one another as expected, that intuition might just be the reason you order an additional IHC that steers you away from misdiagnosis.

B. Workflow Optimization

Prioritize critical or complex cases during peak focus hours.	For example, look at a series of lymph nodes in the morning when your energy reserves are full, as saving these for later in the day risks overlooking that subcapsular cell cluster due to mental fatigue and inadvertent inattention.
Use checklists for case completion, including pending stains or reviews.	Sticky notes are your friends. I paste them onto the slide trays themselves to remind me what is pending, what I must do to finalize the case, etc. This, paired with case triage, is the key to efficiency in the pathology department.

C. Communication and Professional Growth

Document meticulously; clarity is kindness to your future self (and colleagues).	In complex cases or cases that necessitate multiple rounds of ancillary tests, record your findings and questions as you go. It's not uncommon to get a third round of stains back, forgetting exactly what features of the 40-slide case made you order them in the first place and what your diagnostic question was. Mark your slides, write down your questions for the case, and even if not common practice for your specific subspecialty, jot down a microscopic description so that when you return to the case after receiving ancillary studies, you remember the features of the entity that required discernment.
Network and collaborate: learn from techs, assistants, staff, and other residents.	Every laboratory staff member has skills and aptitudes that you do not. By being kind, helpful, and collegiate, others will be more willing to help you when you have questions that cross into their realm of expertise. Especially with gross examinations, respect the pathologists' assistant – learn from them and readily take their advice. I can't count how many times I have relied on their skills and eyesight to complete a case safely and efficiently!

D. Wellness

Embrace 'not knowing' as normal; ask questions early and often.	It is better to ask questions that might seem 'fundamental' early on, as this is when you are building your foundation. Don't neglect general pathologic principles (read Robbins!), as these ground all other learning in pathology and act as a scaffold to understand complex cases and their disease mechanisms. See the things you 'don't know' as opportunities to learn them, not as strikes against your intellect. You are not omniscient– you cannot acquire knowledge simply by willing it into existence!

Appendix D: Resident 'Toolbox': Quick Reference

Before diving into these resources, it's important to recognize that the following compilation of resources isn't exhaustive, nor should it be treated as a mandated curriculum to work through linearly. These are materials I've curated over several years of residency—websites, textbooks, journals, and practical references that I found valuable at different stages of my training (which is still evolving). Some resources overlap significantly in content or focus, so don't feel compelled to consult every item, or become overwhelmed by the breadth displayed here. Instead, use this list as a starting point: explore a few, see which ones resonate with your learning style, and let your day-to-day cases, questions, and interests guide your deeper dives.

A Practical 'Starter Kit' Framework:

- **Robbins and Cotran Pathologic Basis of Disease** should be your foundational reference. It's the gold standard for understanding general pathology and is essential for both exam preparation and day-to-day diagnostic reasoning.
- Pair this with a solid **normal histology reference** (e.g., Histology for Pathologists or, my favourite as a beginning pathology resident, Histology: A Text and Atlas by Pawlina). Understanding 'normal' is the gateway to confidently recognizing the abnormal.
- For a deeper or organ-specific study, add **Sternberg's Diagnostic Surgical Pathology**. This is big general surgical pathology

N. Pardell, *Scalpel, Scope, and Stain*,
https://doi.org/10.1007/978-3-032-25384-2

textbook organized by organs, and great for expanding your diagnostic differentials or tackling rare cases.

- For quick lookups, images, and concise diagnostic criteria, regularly use a reputable online resource like **PathologyOutlines**. It's ideal for rapid referencing in the resident room, especially when you need a synopsis or a photomicrograph in a hurry.

Ultimately, let these resources serve you—not the other way around. The key is not consuming everything, but rather finding what helps you learn and retain most effectively. Let your evolving workflow and the cases in front of you determine which tools become your favourites.

Websites

A. **General Pathology, Surgical Pathology and Case Archives**
  - **PathologyOutlines** (https://www.pathologyoutlines.com/)
  - Free, frequently updated reference/textbook with quick facts, diagnostic criteria, and images. Also lists many fellowships and other resources for all things pathology.
  - **LibrePathology** (https://librepathology.org/wiki/Main_Page)
  - Open-source, community-driven articles on all major domains. Check out the 'An introduction to pathology' page when starting out!
  - **WebPathology** (https://www.webpathology.com/)
  - Extensive digital slide collection with diagnostic notes.
  - **PathPrimer/ExpertPath** (https://app.pathprimer.com/, https://app.expertpath.com/)
  - Comprehensive diagnostic reference (subscription required).
  - **Merck Manuals Professional Version** (https://www.merckmanuals.com/professional)
  - Concise clinical and pathologic summaries. Great for reviewing medical diseases.
  - **PathElective** (https://www.pathelective.com/)
  - Free e-learning (cases, lectures, micro and gross images).
  - **MGH PathCast** (https://learn.mghpathology.org/index.php/pathCast)

- Live/archived video lectures by subspecialty; highly regarded, free.
- Subspecialty series (Breast, Cytopathology, GI, GU, Neuro, Heme, Peds, Gyne, Derm, Head and Neck, etc.)
- **ARUP Laboratories Video Lectures** (University of Utah) (https://arup.utah.edu/education/videoIndex.php)
- Extensive free video lectures and archived content for anatomic and clinical pathology; broad subspecialty coverage.
- **Pathology Learning Centre (UCT)** (https://health.uct.ac.za/pathology-learning-centre)
- Gross/pathological specimen images, digital pathology, teaching resources, virtual slides
- **University of Leeds Virtual Microscopy** (https://www.virtualpathology.leeds.ac.uk/)
- Publicly available histology teaching slides (virtual microscope).
- **Virtual Microscopy Database** (https://www.virtualmicroscopydatabase.org/home)

B. **Subspecialty**
  - **TheAutopsyBook** (https://theautopsybook.com/)
  - Modern autopsy techniques, protocols, and best practices.
  - **Pathways and Diagrams by Disease Area (Cell Signalling Technology)** (https://www.cellsignal.com/pathways/by-disease-area)
  - Curated diagrams/pathways for signalling and disease processes, including Hallmarks of Cancer, autoimmunity, fibrosis, and many more

C. **Reference Institutions/Organizations**
  - **WHO Blue Books Tumour Classifications Online** (https://tumourclassification.iarc.who.int/welcome/)
  - Gold-standard reference for tumour typing (institutional/personal subscription). Has print copies of each book for the physically inclined.
  - **CAP (College of American Pathologists)** (https://www.cap.org/)

- All guidelines, protocols, reporting synoptics, checklists, educational activities, & news.
- **CAP-ACP (Canadian Association of Pathologists)** (https://cap-acp.org/default.aspx)
- Canadian standards, education, and advocacy.

D. **Education/Question Banks**
- **ASCP Resident Question Bank** (https://www.ascp.org/)
- Practice questions, board prep, and review.
- **PathPrimer** (https://app.pathprimer.com/)
- Practice questions (in addition to the diagnostic references noted above)
- **Pathology Journals** (Seek out major *review articles*, especially for up-to-date evidence-based summaries on common and rare entities)
- Modern Pathology
- Histopathology
- American Journal of Surgical Pathology
- Archives of Pathology & Laboratory Medicine
- Acta Neuropathologica
- Annual Review of Pathology: Mechanisms of Disease

Textbooks

A. **General Pathology**
- **Robbins and Cotran Pathologic Basis of Disease**—Foundational textbook.
- **Robbins Basic Pathology**—Concise, abridged version of the above for high yield learning.

B. **Surgical Pathology/Organ-based**
- **Diagnostic Surgical Pathology (Mills and Sternberg)**
- **Ace my Path Series** (https://www.acemypath.com/)
- **Surgical Pathology Reimagined (Gupta)**—Organ-specific, high-yield, case-driven, with photomicrographs and gross images.

- **The Practice of Surgical Pathology: A Beginner's Guide to the Diagnostic Process (Molavi)**—Practical, perfect for new trainees.
- **Differential Diagnosis in Surgical Pathology (Gattuso)**
- **The Washington Manual of Hematopathology (Abro)**
- **Molecular Surgical Pathology (Cheng)**

C. **Frozen Section and Intraoperative Consultation**
- **Frozen Section Pathology: Diagnostic Challenges**
- **Biopsy Interpretation: The Frozen Section**

D. **Autopsy**
- **The Hospital Autopsy (Diagnostic Pathology Series)**
- **Autopsy Pathology: A Manual and Atlas** – Stepwise approach with detailed images.

E. **Cytopathology**
- **Cytology—Diagnostic Principles and Clinical Correlates (Cibas)**
- **Quick Reference Handbook for Surgical Pathologists (includes cytologic pearls) (Rekhtman)**

F. **Normal Histology**
- **Histology: A Text and Atlas (Pawlina)**
- **Normal Histology (Lindberg)**—Excellent normal reference.
- **Histology for Pathologists (Mills)**—Detailed normal micro-anatomical reference with direct comparisons to relevant pathologic findings.

G. **Forensic Pathology**
- **Forensic Pathology (DiMaio)**—Definitive, go-to text reference
- **Forensic Medicine (Simpson)**—Core forensic reference.
- **Forensic and Clinical Forensic Autopsy: An Atlas and Handbook (Pomara)**

Final Encouragement

Starting pathology can feel like restarting medical education due to learning things never taught in medical school, and being exposed to all the processes that make a laboratory functional. But with persistence and a curious mind, the knowledge comes faster than you think. Keep a positive outlook—everyone feels this way when they start! By making it into residency, you've shown aptitude and prowess in learning, traits that are required and indispensable in this specialty. In diagnostics, the learning never ends, and just because you might have a Royal College certification at the end of the training program does not mean you've learned it all. This is truly a gift—a profession and occupation that never grows stale, always surprises you with wonder, and always has a profound impact on patient care. Stay collegial, affable, compassionate, and meticulous, and everything else will fall into place.

N. Pardell, *Scalpel, Scope, and Stain*,
https://doi.org/10.1007/978-3-032-25384-2

Index

N. Pardell, *Scalpel, Scope, and Stain*,
https://doi.org/10.1007/978-3-032-25384-2

FSC
www.fsc.org
MIX
Papier | Fördert
gute Waldnutzung
FSC® C083411

Zeitfracht Medien GmbH
Ferdinand-Jühlke-Straße 7
99095 Erfurt, Deutschland
produktsicherheit@kolibri360.de